Marathon *of* Faith

Marathon
of Faith

REX AND JANET LEE
WITH JIM BELL

DESERET BOOK COMPANY
SALT LAKE CITY, UTAH

Photograph on page 20 by Mish Studio, Mesa, Arizona. Photo on page 32 by John Metelsky, National Press Club, Washington, D.C. Photo on page 64 by Doug Martin. Photos on pages 78, 100, 140, 188, 189, 192 (top) by Mark Philbrick. Photos on pages 119, 190 (top), 191 (bottom), and back cover jacket by Merrett Smith. Photo on page 118 by Don Busath. Photos on page 185 by BYU Photo Studio (Rex in mid-1950s) and Foto Herman, Mexico (Janet in mid-1950s). Photo on page 192 (bottom) by Patricia Evans. Photo on page 194 (bottom) by Dave Newman Photography.

© 1996 Janet G. Lee and James P. Bell

Library of Congress Cataloging-in-Publication Data

Lee, Rex E., 1935–1996.
    Marathon of faith / by Rex & Janet Lee, with Jim Bell.
        p.   cm.
    ISBN 1-57345-163-0
    1. Lee, Rex E., 1935–1996—Health. 2. Lymphoma—Patients—United States—Biography. I. Lee, Janet, 1938–   . II. Bell, Jim, 1952–   .
III. Title.
RC280.L9L425   1996
362.1'9699442'0092—dc20
[B]   96-10450
                                                                        CIP

Printed in the United States of America

10   9   8   7   6   5   4   3   2   1

To our children—Diana, Tom, Wendy,
Michael, Stephanie, Melissa, and Christie

If suffering alone taught,
all the world would be wise.

—ANNE MORROW LINDBERGH

CONTENTS

PREFACE

In 1987, at a time when our lives were filled with richness and joy, we learned early one morning that Rex had cancer. There had been some indications that something was wrong—most of which we had overlooked—but nothing, it seemed at the time, could have prepared us for this news.

Over the next several months, Rex and I joined together in battling this illness, and for a time it appeared we had won. Then in 1990, just six months after Rex became president of Brigham Young University, a second cancer was diagnosed, which was followed by several other medical challenges.

A few weeks before the discovery of Rex's second cancer, we had given a devotional talk at BYU in which we shared some of the details of Rex's battle with cancer, as well as some of the lessons we had drawn from that experience. Soon after, it was suggested that we ought to share our experiences more fully in the form of a book, and at different times after that talk similar suggestions were made.

Rex, in particular, felt that perhaps sharing our experiences might have some value to others, and in July 1995 we finally began in earnest to prepare our story for publication. Had we known then what was ahead for us, we might have been hesitant to commit to writing this book. But as the manuscript neared completion and as Rex's health deteriorated, he, in particular, felt a strong desire to complete the project.

This book, however, is not a book about cancer, although our particular challenges came in that form. Rather, it is a book about the joy that can be found in all of life, whether we are living amidst the pains or the pleasures of mortality. Our experiences suggest that joy exists not around the edges of our challenges—where we may find a temporary release—but at the very core and center of adversity.

Our desire in sharing our story has been to convey something of the universality of suffering, which binds together all of humanity in ways that our individual pleasures cannot. Of course, we have been well aware that countless individuals and families have faced and will yet face challenges far more severe and shattering than ours. Our hope has been that there might be some value in sharing with broader circles something of what we all experience in uniquely individual ways and that such sharing is one way of helping lift one another's burdens.

This book makes no attempt to serve as a biography. Much more could have been said about Rex's service in government, for example, or his years at BYU, but we have left out many, many details and experiences in order to focus primarily on the challenges we have faced.

During the writing of the manuscript, we often found it difficult to decide what events to include, but more of a challenge was deciding *whom* to include. Throughout the nine years of our challenges, our lives literally were blessed daily by the thoughtful acts of countless individuals. Yet each time we named a doctor who had gone to great lengths to help Rex, we would think of five more who had rendered similar compassion and service. And each time we mentioned an act of kindness performed by a family member or friend, we would remember dozens more whose concern was manifested in equally significant ways. At different points in our writing, we discussed the possibility of leaving out all names, thus avoiding the appearance that one person's thoughtfulness meant more to us than another's, but in the end we realized that some names were needed to carry the story forward.

So to our many friends and associates who were, indeed, a part of this story but whose names do not appear in print—neighbors, ward members, professional colleagues, doctors, nurses, therapists, technicians, hospital staff, university students, friends, and family members who helped us see more clearly the blessings of our eternal connectedness—we would simply say that we have thanked our Heavenly Father countless times for your never-ending kindnesses and hope you will understand this acknowledgement of your generous service.

In preparing this book, we have likewise appreciated the help of individuals too numerous to mention, but we do feel a need to recognize the efforts of at least a few, including Sheri Dew, vice president of publishing at Deseret Book, who persisted over several years in trying to convince us that ours is a story worth telling; Jim Bell, who helped us arrange the journals, talks, interviews, random notes, and discussions that helped to form this book; Janet Calder and Jan Nelson, Rex's secretaries at BYU, who helped in countless ways as we prepared this manuscript; Linda Gundry and Michelle Eckersley of Deseret Book, who, respectively, edited and designed the book, with sensitivity and insight; and our children and children-in-law, who refreshed our memories, offered editorial suggestions, and supported us during the preparation of the manuscript, as well as through all that we have undergone.

—*Janet Lee*
March 1996

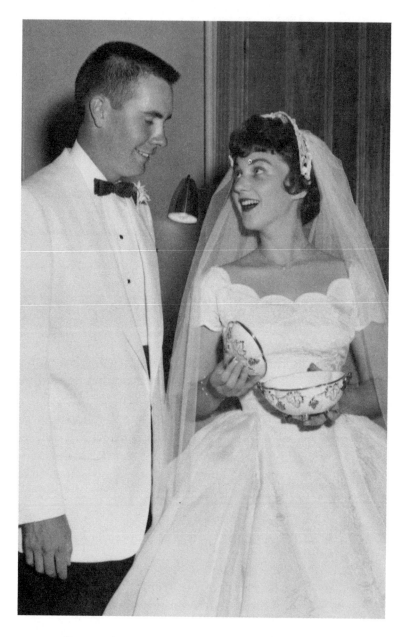

REX AND JANET ON THEIR WEDDING DAY, JULY 7, 1959

INTRODUCTION

Rex Lee is by any standard a remarkable man—founding dean of a law school, United States assistant attorney general and then solicitor general, and president of Brigham Young University, to name some of the titles that suggest the broad scope of his success. And, like many men and women of accomplishment, he grew up in a small town.

Born February 27, 1935, he grew up in St. Johns, Arizona. Rex recalls that there was only one paved road through town until his late high school years and that open irrigation ditches lined with poplar trees and green grass flowed along the streets, providing a grazing area for the cows that freely roamed the streets prior to the town's incorporation.

The town's schools were small and the teachers few, but each was personally acquainted with the students and their families—and took a personal interest in each pupil's progress. Young Rex showed considerable potential, and the teachers pushed him to excel. (His mother recalls having to push him to set aside his schoolwork and go out to play). He also learned much from his family, who owned one of the town's grocery stores as well as a sawmill business in which he spent his summers from the time he was eight years old until he was in law school.

Working in the sawmills, which were located in Arizona and New Mexico, provided Rex with a variety of learning experiences and helped him see the caliber of men his father and other relatives were. He remembers well one summer when the ward in a neighboring town was building a chapel and ordered a shipment of boards twenty-four feet in length, rather than the standard sixteen-foot lengths the mill normally produced. This change in specifications added to the expense of the lumber, and when Rex's father and grandfather attempted to negotiate a higher price, the bishop refused to pay. The matter was then submitted for arbitration to the Church building department, which decided in favor of the sawmill. But when the transaction was over, Rex later learned, his father and grandfather sent a contribution to the ward exceeding the difference the mill had been paid.

Throughout his life, Rex has joked that the local Baskin-Robbins ice cream store only had two flavors and that he was sixteen before he discovered that the name of his town was not "Resume Speed." But he also knows, in his words, that "a very large part of what I am I owe to that little nineteenth-century Mormon settlement in which I was raised."

Half a world away, as Rex was learning to read, Janet Griffin was born to Marian and Ben Griffin in Paris, France, where Ben was an entry-level clerk with the American embassy. Soon after Janet's birth, as the first rumblings of war were being heard across Europe, the family was evacuated from Paris aboard the last commercial ship to leave France before the outbreak of World War II. When Ben was later drafted and sent back to

Europe, Marian and her three small children moved to Ogden, Utah, near both her and Ben's family.

When Marian, together with her children and parents-in-law, returned home after taking Ben to the train station, Marian remembers that "Ben's mother broke down under the pressure of sending her son off to war. I had been trying to be courageous, especially in front of Janet and her brother, Glen, but when my mother-in-law began crying, I went into my room to get my own emotions under control. Soon after, Janet came in and held my hand to help me feel better, but I was still overcome with emotion. After a few minutes she said, 'Mom, we can't let Grandmother see us cry. Daddy used to be her little boy, and we need to be brave for her.'"

Janet's father returned safely, and when the family finally was reunited, they moved to New Jersey, where Ben resumed his work with the United States Treasury Department in New York City.

During the summer after second grade, Janet began to feel unusually tired and was plagued with a constant cough. Soon she became so weak that she sometimes asked her father to carry her on family outings. Her condition grew worse, and soon the family's doctor had Janet's parents take her to a nearby hospital for tests. As the seven-year-old girl stood waiting to be X-rayed, she noticed that the woman in front of her was crying. Thinking the tears were caused by fear for what was about to happen and wanting very much to help, Janet took her hand and said, "Don't worry, the machine won't hurt you." When her illness was finally diagnosed as tuberculosis, the doctors wanted to admit her to a tuberculosis sanitarium in New York, but her parents felt she was too young to be that far away from her family. So for the next six months, Janet was confined to her bed at home, where her mother cared for her.

Not long after Janet's recovery, her mother became very ill with asthma and one day lapsed into a state of unconsciousness. Janet watched as Marian was taken away in an ambulance and then went for weeks without being able to visit her mother because children weren't allowed in the hospital. Marian's condition necessitated a move to a climate more conducive to her health, and soon Janet, together with her brother and three-year-old sister, went to the airport to see her off and then waited while her father sold their house and made the arrangements to move to El Paso, Texas.

Even though the family had moved several times before Janet was a teenager, there was a constancy in the Griffin home as the family ate breakfast and dinner together each day and engaged in thoughtful discussions on world events, the children's education, and spiritual concerns. The family also camped and attended operas and symphonies together, and Janet was able to travel with her father on short business trips, where they would talk as they traveled, ate together, and attended to Ben's responsibilities with the U.S. Treasury Department. From a very young age, Janet enjoyed an interesting mix of family fun coupled with the world of politics, diplomacy, and formal entertaining.

Meanwhile, Rex grew up riding horses and going to rodeos in the rural world of St. Johns. As he looked toward his future, he thought fleetingly, as boys often do, of becoming a pilot or a cowboy, but by his sophomore year in high school, he had set his sights on becoming a lawyer.

When the time came for him to go away to college—and being from St. Johns, he had no choice but to go away to college—his science and English teachers counseled him to attend the University of Arizona and suggested that he could likely receive the prestigious Phelps Dodge Scholarship if he would apply. Rex's parents, on the other hand, wanted him to attend Brigham Young University in Provo, Utah. The family finally reached an agreement that he would try BYU for one year and then transfer to the University of Arizona if he didn't like it. So in the fall of 1953, he and three friends loaded their belongings into a 1943 Chevrolet and made the 600-mile trip to Provo, Utah, driving at a top speed of fifty miles per hour.

They arrived in Provo late at night, where they had signed

up to live in one of the D-Dorms—seven army barracks that had been converted to student housing. But the supply office for their dormitory was closed, so while they were able to get into their rooms, they had no mattresses, no sheets, no blankets, no pillows, and no electricity. Rex later recalled:

> *Though they made my situation a bit more bleak, those slight inconveniences were not at the heart of the discouragement I felt. My world seemed to be closing in around me, and my outlook was as dark as the room I occupied. Here I was, 600 miles away from home, and about to become a member of a freshman class three and a half times the size of the total population of my hometown, and full of misgivings about whether a boy from St. Johns could make it at a big university.*
>
> *Instinctively, I got down on my knees, put my elbows on the wire mesh that served as the springs for my unmattressed bed, and began some of the most earnest pleading with my Heavenly Father that I had ever undertaken.*
>
> *It helped. I felt that I was not alone, that I had a partner who was interested in me and willing to help. Though my earthly parents were located hundreds of miles to the south, my Heavenly Father was very much there with me. And while my misgivings did not completely disappear, the stifling discouragement gave way to a healthy anxiety.*

Rex decided after one quarter that BYU was where he wanted to complete his undergraduate education. After finishing his first two years of college, he accepted a calling to serve as a missionary in what was then known as the Mexican Mission of The Church of Jesus Christ of Latter-day Saints. His mission president, Claudius Bowman, took note of the young missionary and called him as one of his counselors in the mission presidency.

Elder Lee was serving in this capacity when President and Sister Bowman's friends Ben and Marian Griffin moved to Mexico City, where Ben was treasury attaché at the United

States embassy. As it was Christmastime, their daughter Janet, who was in her first term at BYU, accompanied them. Her boyfriend from El Paso, Texas, was with them. President Bowman offered to drive the Griffins around the city as they looked for a place to stay, and the Griffin family divided into two groups riding in two separate cars—one driven by President Bowman, the other by his counselor, Elder Lee.

Quite by chance, Janet and her boyfriend ended up in the second car, and while she paid no particular attention to the elder driving, he certainly noticed her. In fact, he adjusted his rearview mirror so that he could keep an eye on her as they drove through the streets of residential Mexico City. Janet returned to BYU, but as her parents got to know Elder Lee during their months in Mexico, they sometimes mentioned him in their calls and letters to her.

Janet had mixed emotions about this missionary she scarcely knew. On the one hand, she found her parents' attempts to pique her interest in Elder Lee a bit annoying. Once, while visiting in Mexico, she responded to someone's suggestion that Elder Lee might look her up at BYU by declaring, "I have heard enough about this 'paragon of virtue,' and I am going to make a public statement. I am not interested in Rex Lee; I will never be interested in Rex Lee; in fact, I don't even know Rex Lee. But I don't think I like him at all."

At another time, however, she attended a district conference with her father, who was a branch president, where Elder Lee spoke. In Janet's words:

> It was a small, crowded chapel where we all sat—
> almost sticking together in the heat of the afternoon. As
> the meeting got underway, my attention was averted to a
> young mother trying to manage her restless children.
> When she tried to feed them tortillas to quiet them, I was
> amused at the sameness of children everywhere.
> Given my limited Spanish, I knew listening to the
> meeting and understanding would be an effort, as well as

a good exercise, but when Elder Lee spoke, I found myself comprehending most of his flowing and flawless Spanish. As I watched and listened, I felt a unity with his spiritual convictions. The goodness of his character and the simple sincerity of his dedication to what he believed—and what I, too, believed—was evident in every word he spoke. I was momentarily mesmerized, forgetting my dislike for him. For a split second, I thought he was speaking directly to me, and I wondered if we would meet again.

The first day Rex was back at BYU after his mission was a rainy March morning in 1958, and as he ran across the campus he bumped into a young girl who was partially hidden by her umbrella. The two students looked at each other with a vague sense of familiarity, but neither spoke a word. That night it occurred to Rex that this girl might be Brother Griffin's daughter Janet. He called her and asked if she was the person he had run into earlier that day. When she answered yes, he asked her out for Friday night, but she told him she already had a date. When he asked her out for Saturday, he received the same response. There was a long pause, during which Janet recalled both her previous experience and a letter from her mother, extolling Elder Lee's virtues and indicating that she hoped he would call Janet. She also remembered these words from the letter: "You don't have to marry the guy, but I love him. So at least be nice if he calls."

As Rex remembers the story, Janet finally broke the silence by doing something she had never done before—she encouraged her caller to ask again, telling him that she didn't have a date for Sunday. His first thought was to say, "Well, let me know how you come out on getting one." But he swallowed his pride and asked her to go with him to church.

Janet and Rex's first date was rocky, at best. She remembers that he spent a good part of the evening telling her why the person she was then dating was all wrong for her—and then he followed up by encouraging her to change her major.

The romance of Rex and Janet may have had an uneasy beginning, but Janet recognized very early that Rex had great spiritual and intellectual depth. She was always aware of Rex's unusual enthusiasm and began to be captivated by his very contagious personality. She knew after very few encounters with Rex that he was a leader and a steadfast member of the Church. His charm, integrity, and confidence was intriguing and invigorating. She enjoyed the way Rex loved live, worked hard, and knew how to have a good time. Janet remembers being at a college dance, surrounded by Rex's friends from Arizona. She noted that the young man she could picture still as a missionary in Mexico, wearing a slightly wrinkled suit, was now wearing Levi's and seemed to effortlessly capture the attention of the entire crowd. In a few short, simple moments, she knew she was falling in love with Rex Lee.

In Janet's eyes their relationship blended the best of Camelot and the Garden of Eden. "I am so very, very much in love," she wrote to her younger sister, Lois, during her engagement, "and every day I learn new things about Rex that make me love him more and more. I can just imagine the kind of life we will have together. We will have a perfect marriage, perfect children, and a perfect life. Our hearts will know eternal joy."

She was the romantic in this relationship, with idealistic views about how their life would unfold. At one point in their engagement she suggested that they should decide how many children they would have—and what their names would be. Although Rex had his own kind of drive and determination, his feeling was that they should take at least that part of their life one step at a time.

Rex and Janet were married on July 7, 1959, in the Mesa Arizona Temple, and Rex's matter-of-fact practicality immediately surfaced as, on the third day of their honeymoon, he awoke Janet with the romantic reminder that she needed to complete three correspondence courses before September and that she ought to get up and get going.

Janet finished her degree in three years, knowing that they

would soon be leaving Provo so Rex could attend law school. When both of them graduated from BYU in 1960, the Lees moved to Chicago, where he attended the University of Chicago Law School and she taught elementary school for one year in a Chicago suburb and the next two years at the University of Chicago Laboratory School.

During his first year of law school, Rex faced what he viewed as a very difficult situation: It seemed that no matter how hard he studied, he would sit through class amazed at the brilliant insights of his classmates. He often found himself thinking, *I wish I had thought of that* when someone made an insightful comment, and he also contemplated the difficulty of making it through law school. He eased his worries somewhat when he came to the simple conclusion that if he was good enough to get into law school, he was good enough to get out.

After three years of hard work, he did get out—with the number-one ranking in his graduating class and a one-year appointment as a law clerk for Justice Byron R. White of the United States Supreme Court.

Rex enjoyed learning of the inner workings of the nation's highest court, and Rex and Janet both enjoyed the excitement of Washington, D.C., where Janet's parents had also moved at about the same time. When Rex's appointment with the Supreme Court ended in 1964, they were both ready to settle down in Arizona, where he had been hired by the Phoenix law firm of Jennings, Strouss, Salmon & Trask. Rex was excited to get back "home" to Arizona, and Janet was thrilled at the prospect of planting lasting roots for the first time in her life. Although she had enjoyed many things about living all over the world with her parents, she wanted her young family— which consisted of their eighteen-month-old daughter, Diana, and another child on the way—to know the stability of a permanent home.

Janet remembers their years in Tempe as near-perfect. She and Rex raised their young family, built a home, and shared in Church service and community activities. Days full of

Arizona's sunshine, happy children, and the completeness of a joyful marriage transformed Janet's life into her Camelot.

Rex was made a partner in his law firm three years after joining, and there was talk in some circles that he might have a political career ahead of him. And while he worked hard at the law, he also worked hard at being a good father and husband. Once, when he took a harsh tone with his daughter Diana, then two and a half years old, she responded by telling him, "Daddy, you shouldn't talk like that to wittle childwens." He took that to heart and tried all the harder to treat his children with respect.

When he came home from work each day, he would lie down in the yet-to-be-furnished living room and, rather than insist on silence, encourage his children to play a game he had invented called "Run around Daddy," the object of which was to circle Rex without getting tripped and then tickled by their father. He notes that by playing this game, he could get a bit of rest while he entertained his children.

Janet particularly enjoyed the almost eight years she and Rex lived in Tempe—which was longer than she had ever lived in one place. In Tempe she found the sense of security and stability she had always hoped for.

When the Lees heard in the spring of 1971 that BYU's board of trustees had announced that the university was going to establish a law school, they found the news to be an interesting topic of conversation, but nothing more than that. Soon, however, Rex was visited by Ernest L. Wilkinson, who was stepping down as president of BYU and was helping establish the law school. The two talked about various LDS lawyers who could serve on the law school faculty, and President Wilkinson asked Rex if he would be willing to come to Salt Lake City to meet with the committee who would select a dean for the school. The committee consisted of Elders Marion G. Romney, Howard W. Hunter, Boyd K. Packer, and Marion D. Hanks; Neal A. Maxwell, who was at that time the Church's commissioner of education; President Wilkinson;

and Dallin H. Oaks, who had just been appointed to succeed President Wilkinson as president of BYU.

Rex made the trip in August, discussing with the committee some possible candidates for the faculty and the school's dean. In October, Rex was invited back to Salt Lake City to meet with the committee. Several weeks later, while Rex was in a meeting with several clients, his secretary called in over the intercom, "Do you want to talk to some guy named Harold Lee from Salt Lake City?" Rex wanted to suggest that she speak that name with a good deal more reverence, but instead he quickly concluded his meeting and returned President Lee's call. Within days he and Janet were flying to Salt Lake City to meet with President Lee, who was a counselor in the First Presidency at the time.

When President Lee asked Rex to serve as the founding dean of the BYU law school, Rex and Janet accepted. Then President Lee gave them some wise counsel they have never forgotten. In their private discussions before meeting with President Lee, Janet and Rex had been concerned about the effect this position, if offered, might have on their family financially. In fact, they had decided they would need to know the salary offered before they could make a decision. But after they had accepted—without even discussing salary with President Lee—the wise counselor said, "Janet, you and Rex are still very young, and you will have many decisions to make in your life together. I just want you to know that, from my perspective at least, it is important never to put a monetary stamp on your decisions. Rex will have many opportunities to serve and to grow, but just remember not to base your choices on monetary issues."

Not long after that meeting, Rex and Janet moved to Provo. The two of them worked together to make a new home for their family as well as to establish, from the ground up, the J. Reuben Clark Law School—curriculum, faculty, students, library, building, and all. It was an undertaking that was later characterized by President Oaks as "roughly comparable to

Rex's competing in a 100-yard dash where, as the starting gun sounded, every other runner was already running full tilt while Rex was lying flat on his back at the starting line. He had to get up, pursue the other runners, and make it a competitive race. And that's what Rex Lee did" (*BYU Today*, July 1989, pp. 24–25).

But before the first class of the law school graduated in 1976, Rex was asked by Edward H. Levi (then the U.S. attorney general and formerly dean of the University of Chicago Law School when Rex had been a student there) to move back to Washington, D.C., to serve as assistant attorney general over the Civil Division of the United States Department of Justice. Rex accepted and served in that position from May 1975 through January 1977, having been granted a leave of absence by the university. His division, made up of some 300 lawyers, handled all the civil suits brought either by or against the United States.

The move to Washington was a challenging one for Janet, in particular, as she longed for the roots she had planted in Tempe and then transplanted to Provo. Even with the challenges, though, she was experiencing what she had sensed when she had first started dating Rex years earlier—that life with him was always going to be an adventure.

With the presidential election of 1976 came a new administration, and immediately after Jimmy Carter moved into the White House, the Lees moved back to their home in Provo, where Rex resumed his responsibilities as dean of the law school.

He was only forty-two at the time, and Janet felt that he had done more in those years than most people do in a lifetime. She knew, however, that his accomplishments were not the result of any master plan or list of goals that he had drawn up as a college student. Rather, his one underlying objective was to work as hard as he could at whatever he was doing— and to enjoy what he was doing to the fullest extent possible.

Often, as he tried to get done in a day all the things he felt he needed to, he would end up doing three or four things at once—reviewing a legal brief while he talked on the phone with a faculty member while one of his children hit him up for lunch money. Janet would sometimes try to convince him that even when he covered the phone with his hand, the other party could hear him say, "Good grief, Wendy, I gave you five dollars yesterday!" But it was hard for him to set one thing aside to attend to another, because he knew he could accomplish more by doing both simultaneously.

Janet sometimes tried to convince him to take a little more time off than he was inclined to, but he resisted. Instead of taking the leisurely vacations Janet envisioned, the family would often accompany Rex across the country during the summer months as he taught bar review courses, and he and Janet would take the children to amusement parks when Rex's schedule permitted.

The fall of 1980 brought another shift in the nation's leadership, as Ronald Reagan defeated Jimmy Carter to become the fortieth president of the United States. Not long after, there was talk in some circles that Rex was a likely candidate for the office of solicitor general of the United States, and at about the same time Janet felt strongly that the family was headed back to Washington. The issue, for her, wasn't what position he would be asked to assume but rather how a move would affect the family. She felt strongly enough about her premonition that she started suggesting to the children that they not make any long-term commitments at the schools they were then attending.

Rex's nomination came in May 1981, and he immediately came under attack by congressional Democrats, the National Organization for Women, and other lobbying groups for his opposition to the Equal Rights Amendment, which many groups were struggling to have ratified as part of the United States Constitution. Although the Senate confirmation hearings on solicitors general rarely get noticed beyond the Washington beltway, Rex's hearings made more than the average splash in national headlines as opponents attempted to defeat his nomination to the office that argues all government cases before the United States Supreme Court. Rex stood his ground before the Senate Judiciary Committee, however, and was confirmed in July by the full Senate.

Six of the Lee's children—Tom, Wendy, Michael, Stephanie, Melissa, and Christie—made the move to McLean, Virginia, while their oldest daughter, Diana, stayed in Provo to begin her studies at BYU. Knowing that Tom would soon be starting college too, Janet felt the need to work full-time. She found a job teaching kindergarten at the school Melissa attended. Christie attended preschool there, and Stephanie and Michael rode the bus from their school to Janet's on early-release day so they could help clean chalkboards and start their own homework, all under Janet's supervision. Tom and Wendy drove over to help Janet when their school day was over, too. This system worked well for the Lees, who found that the principal of the private school where Janet taught was both intrigued by and patient with Janet and Rex's large family.

The children had time to play and take piano or dance lessons after they returned home with Janet. Everyone then helped with dinner, dishes, laundry, and homework. Family members were blessed with excellent health; Janet recalls that she left school only twice during those five years to pick up a child who was ill and needed to check out of school. Weekends were usually family time, with Sundays being reserved entirely for Church and family.

On Friday nights the family generally would gather on the couch and play games or watch a movie together, often with the children watching intently while Rex and Janet dozed off behind them. On Saturdays, Rex and Janet had time alone together as they ran along the Potomac River and talked about his cases, her teaching, and each of their children. They would return home from their run for a day of shopping and house-cleaning. (Janet always enjoyed the shocked looks on neighbors' faces as the United States solicitor general opened the door with one hand, while holding the vacuum cleaner in the other.) Then, in the evenings, they would cook out and entertain themselves with a variety of games and activities.

In August 1981, not long after the family's move to Virginia, Rex and Janet received a telephone call from their oldest daughter, Diana, who had stayed behind in Provo to attend BYU. Diana announced her engagement and her plans for a December wedding. Janet, in particular, was stunned. She could not conceive of putting together a wedding reception on top of teaching, taking care of the other six children, and supporting a very busy husband. But more than those considerations, she could not imagine having reached that stage in life at which she would have a married daughter, not to mention a son-in-law.

But as always, Janet managed beautifully. On December 29, Diana married Steven Allred, and the Lees hosted a reception in Provo. Rex and Janet enjoyed seeing all their friends from Provo at the reception, many of whom stayed late into the evening to talk. One, in particular, stayed longer than most—the Lees' family doctor, Lyman Moody. Lyman and Rex were close friends and running partners, and Lyman thought he ought to let Janet know, before she and Rex returned to Washington, that after having run blood tests while the Lees were in town, he continued to feel concern about Rex's low count of white blood cells, which help the body fight off infections. There was no cause for alarm, Lyman explained to Janet, but knowing that she often worried about Rex more than he worried about himself, Lyman thought she ought to be kept current on the situation.

A low white count notwithstanding, Rex returned to Washington and to the frenetic pace he had pursued his whole life. The vagueness of his doctor's suggestion that they watch his white count didn't fit with his mindset that if there's something you can do about a problem, you do it; if there isn't, you don't waste a lot of time worrying about it. Besides, he was in peak physical health, having run twelve marathons in the preceding three years.

In 1982, as Rex was nearing the end of his first year as solicitor general, he was working to bring his old friend Terry Crapo back to Washington as his chief deputy. The two had first known each other as freshmen at BYU, and their lives had followed parallel courses ever since. They both pursued the same major, they took the same classes, they served together in student government (Rex as student body president, with Terry as his executive assistant), they went to law school at the same time (although Terry went to Harvard), and their children were very close in age. Now, for the first time, it appeared that they would have the opportunity to work together professionally.

Then in July, Rex talked with Terry for the last time. Rex's old friend had called to say that he had just found out he had leukemia and that he was going to be admitted to LDS Hospital in Salt Lake City for treatment. When Rex asked how serious his condition was, Terry told him that the doctors were hoping they could get him to the point where they could perform a bone marrow transplant. Rex knew then that his friend's condition was very serious indeed.

Each day for the next several days, Rex called the hospital to get an update on Terry's condition. And each day the news got worse. When Rex called on the tenth day, he learned that Terry had died five minutes earlier.

Rex had dealt several times with the deaths of people close to him, but Terry's passing hit him harder than any other he had ever experienced. Terry, one of his best friends, had been taken in the prime of his life. With Terry's death, Rex realized just how completely unpredictable life can be—and how quickly it can be lost.

Rex's work as solicitor general gave him the opportunity to argue thirty-one cases before the Supreme Court, and his office's win record of almost 80 percent earned it a reputation in legal circles as "the winningest little law firm in

Washington." At home, he enjoyed being involved in his children's lives and helped them with homework, projects, problems, and anything else that he could. And he and Janet were moving comfortably toward the twenty-five-year mark in their marriage.

By 1985, Rex and Janet had decided that four years was about as long as he wished to serve as solicitor general. Upon announcing his resignation, he was besieged with offers from law firms who sought his services, and he ultimately accepted an offer from the large national firm of Sidley & Austin. On July 1, 1985, he became a partner in the Washington office, with his primary focus being appellate cases. That decision was difficult in at least one sense: it meant he would be giving up his longtime association with BYU's law faculty. Feeling that Rex owed his longtime colleagues and the university administration an explanation of the course he had chosen, he and Janet traveled to Provo and met with President Jeffrey R. Holland; the university's provost, Jae R. Ballif; and Carl S. Hawkins, dean of the law school. The three listened politely as Rex explained why he would not be returning to BYU for several years, but then President Ballif surprised Rex by telling him that the university would have no problem with his splitting his time between the BYU law school and his private practice, as long as the Lees would live in Provo. It was ultimately determined that Rex and Janet would spend one more year with their family in Washington as Rex established his relationship with Sidley & Austin, after which time they would move back to Provo. There Rex would rejoin the BYU law faculty and at the same time practice law with his new firm— with the aid of telephones, faxes, and airplanes.

By 1986, when Rex and Janet moved back to Provo, they had come a long way together. He had never imagined, as a boy growing up in St. Johns, that he would one day walk the corridors of power in his country's capital as a regular advocate before its highest court. And while Janet knew full well just how bright and capable her husband was, she had not imagined all that their life together would entail, particularly since she had enthusiastically embraced his original plan of settling in Arizona and practicing law there for the rest of his life. Without question, their journey together had taken some unexpected detours, yet there was a certain constancy amid all the change.

During their first two summers together, Rex had worked in his family's sawmills to earn money for college. One day, half in jest, he asked Janet if she would still love him if he were going to spend the rest of his life in the sawmill camps. Instinctively, she said yes and explained that the work he did had nothing to do with how she felt about him.

A quarter of a century later, Janet was accustomed to the periodic and unpredictable upheavals in the Lee family's lives, and she admired all that he had accomplished as one of the nation's leading lawyers. But as they anticipated settling back into life in Provo, she did so knowing that all Rex had done professionally had nothing to do with the love they shared so personally.

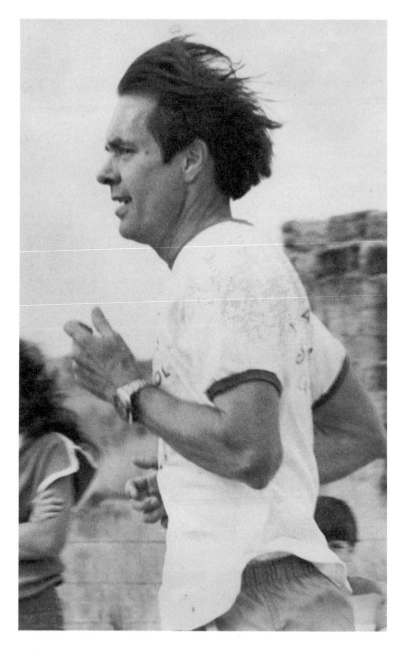

REX COMPETING IN A MARATHON. WHILE SERVING AS DEAN OF BYU'S
J. REUBEN CLARK LAW SCHOOL, REX TOOK UP THE SPORT OF RUNNING;
HE ULTIMATELY COMPLETED THIRTEEN MARATHONS.

CHAPTER 1

A Run along the Potomac

Rex: Following my term as the United States solicitor general, I embarked on what was probably the most challenging, exciting, and stressful period of my life. In June 1985 I joined the law firm of Sidley & Austin and began to rebuild a full-time, private legal practice—an arena in which I had not worked since coming to BYU as founding dean of the law school in 1971.

Much of my work involved arguing cases before the United States Supreme Court, the first step of which involves submitting a writ of certiorari—a written brief outlining the reasons why a given case should be considered by the Court. The second step—and this part of the process is not taught in law school—is waiting for the Court's answer. In general, the Court accepts only about 2 percent of the cases presented at this first stage; and those odds, combined with the weeks of waiting, created within me some anxiety each time I waited for the Court's listing of the cases it would hear.

For at least a couple of days before the Court's announcement, I would be filled with anticipation. It was amazing what a disparity in my level of happiness could result from one of two simple words, spoken by a Supreme Court clerk over the telephone: "granted" or "denied."

During the spring of 1986, as I awaited notification on one particular case, I was also filled with anticipation over another significant moment in my life: the return of our oldest son, Tom, from his mission in Mexico. I rehearsed over and over in my mind the upcoming event as I pictured my family waiting at the airport gate and then imagined my son stepping into view. I wondered how he would look—heavier, thinner, older? And, more important, I wondered what changes I would come to see inside of my son.

It was my good fortune that, within a ten-day period, the Supreme Court agreed to hear our case—and my son arrived home as scheduled. All of our children except Diana were with Janet and me at the Washington National Airport, and when Tom finally emerged from the plane, I felt a surge of joy upon seeing him after his two-year absence. I was immediately struck by his physical maturity, and in the following weeks I discovered that he had matured spiritually and intellectually as well.

That weekend, Diana came for Tom's homecoming talk, which was the first time in two years that all of our children had been together at the same time. Watching them reminded me of the friendship Janet and I share with each of our children and of the fact that, with the exception of minor skirmishes here and there, they are really quite good friends with each other.

During these months—and as I looked toward the coming year—I had a feeling of complete well-being and contentment. My life at that time was as good as it had ever been. I was running regularly and in excellent health. I was becoming a specialist in Supreme Court cases to an extent that I had never envisioned when I returned to private practice. My relationship with Janet was growing stronger and stronger. And each of our seven children was bringing us great joy as they grew and matured.

Janet: As our last year in the Washington, D.C., area came to a close and we anticipated our return to Utah, our lives were as full and good as they had ever been. When Rex returned to private practice, I had been called almost immediately as the Young Women president in our McLean, Virginia, ward. With our daughters Wendy and Stephanie in that age group, I was excited about the chance to be with my girls and their friends. I have always found that closeness comes from interacting at various levels with my children, and my work in Young Women brought another dimension to our lives as we camped, rehearsed for plays, and shared spiritual experiences.

When we were finally ready to move back to Provo, we felt a wide range of emotions. During our five years in Washington, our family had changed; instead of ranging in age from toddler through teenagers, our children now ranged from grade-schoolers through a returned missionary and a college graduate (who was also a wife and mother). Rex and I had become grandparents, and we had all established strong ties in the Virginia area. We savored the lush Virginia countryside, and we thrived on living so near to the hub of political activity in the nation's capital.

But within days after arriving back in Provo, everyone in the family felt comfortable—as if we were slipping our feet, which were exhausted after a cross-country move, into old bedroom slippers.

As school started in the fall of 1986, all of our children were back in Provo. Tom and Wendy were living in apartments near campus while they attended BYU, but they found countless reasons to drop by for visits—to eat, write papers, watch videos with friends, and talk to us about their lives. On Sundays we always had dinner together, and our children who attended BYU often brought roommates. Diana, our married daughter, was expecting her second child, and her husband, Steve, was attending law school at BYU. Diana and I would often run together, and more than once I said to her that life seemed almost too perfect and that I worried that it couldn't remain that way forever. She cringed the first time I made the comment, but we later discussed my feeling at length, leaving us both uneasy with the premonition that something was going to happen that would change the course of our lives.

This ominous feeling didn't come very often, and I would completely forget about it soon after it did. Life was so good that I, too, was nearly convinced that nothing could stand in the way of our total happiness.

Rex: As the beginning of the school year approached, I had some fears about how well I would handle teaching in the law school and maintaining a law practice, but it didn't take long before I had settled into a routine that seemed to work fine. I made heavy use of the telephone, overnight delivery services, and my fax machine. Working as an appellate specialist, I could do most of my work in my office and schedule courtroom appearances well in advance. This arrangement provided me with enough flexibility that I was able to be a part of the very large Sidley & Austin firm from my one-man office in Provo, Utah.

I also found returning to the classroom to be very gratifying, and in general I enjoyed the excitement that always, at least for me, accompanies the newness and freshness of a change, no matter what it is.

My busyness has both positive and negative aspects but is part of my general nature. I have always tried to use my time for what I view as productive purposes. When I traveled in connection with my law practice, I brought work to do on the plane or in hotel rooms, and I spent my free time doing whatever would keep my professional ball moving down the field. And when I went home at night, my thoughts automatically turned to whether I should be mowing the lawn, washing the dishes, helping children with homework, or running to the store.

I have never liked using the word *compulsive* to describe my nature, but I suppose it does. Relaxing has never come easy to me. Only rarely during those hectic days would I give in to the urge to relax. When I did take time to contemplate, however, I felt good about Janet's and my life in general. As the school year progressed, life couldn't have been better. Our third child, Wendy, was dating her high school boyfriend, Tom Jacobson, who had returned home from his mission not long after our Tom did. My fatherly supposition was that they would be married before long. In addition, Wendy had introduced her brother Tom to her roommate, Kimberly Johnson. I began to be sobered by the thought that within a year we could have not one but three married children. Our younger four children—Michael, Stephanie, Melissa, and Christie—still lived at home, adding vitality and variety to our lives.

In October 1986, I went to Washington again to argue another case before the Supreme Court. This was of particular significance to me because it had been twenty years, almost to the week, since I, as a young Phoenix lawyer, had argued my first case before the nation's highest court. And even though I had been around the track forty times, the night before I presented my argument was the same as all the rest, as I worried whether I should reread the briefs or the pertinent cases themselves or my outline. I agonized over what questions I would be asked, and by which justices. As I sat in my hotel room, I rehearsed the answers I had prepared. After scores of hours of work—sometimes even hundreds—my professional life always came down to this one half-hour oral argument, which begins in each case with "Mr. Chief Justice, and may it please the Court," and ends with "Unless the Court has questions, I have nothing further."

I felt wonderful after arguing the case the next afternoon, even though I would have to wait for several months for the Court's decision. The argument had gone as well as could be expected, and I was also looking forward to what I knew would be a very pleasant vacation with Janet and her family.

Janet: As my sister, brother, and I looked ahead to our parents' fifty-third wedding anniversary, we thought it would be nice for us, our spouses, and our parents to spend a few days together—a rather rare occurrence, given our hectic lives. So we arranged to meet in Carlsbad, California, a quiet coastal town near San Diego. This was the first time in my memory that the eight of us had been together for a vacation without our children, and it led to many interesting discussions and thoughtful moments as we spent five days together enjoying sun, surf, and solitude.

Late one afternoon, my sister, Lois, and I were walking together on the beach, and before long our conversation took a serious turn as we began discussing life, its challenges, and what we perceived as our growing ability to handle whatever came our way.

"I think I have lived long enough now that I could handle any challenge given me," I naively stated to Lois, and she replied, "I think I could too."

Then my sister asked me this question: "Janet, what would be the most difficult challenge you could imagine having to face?"

I didn't even need to think about my answer. I already knew. "I can't imagine life without Rex," I began. "The hardest thing for me would be to lose Rex to a horrible illness."

Lois thought for a minute and then said, "That would be hard, but I think divorce would be even more difficult for me."

We both were immediately struck by the preposterousness of our fears. Rex, after all, was the picture of health. He had run thirteen marathons over the preceding eight years, and he rarely even caught a cold. My sister was entering the twenty-second year of a marriage that seemed intact, and the seriousness of our discussion soon gave way to laughter as we considered suggestions that couldn't possibly become realities.

Rex: As always happens, vacations come to an end. When Janet and I returned to Provo, our lives were as busy as ever. My two jobs were more demanding than I had anticipated, and Janet had commented before we left for Carlsbad that when we got back we were going to need to make some changes so we could slow life down a little.

Well, the change we made was that the very next Sunday I was sustained as bishop of Provo's Oak Hills Third Ward. Interestingly, I had served in the same position in 1978—for a full week, after which time I had been called as president of the BYU Seventh Stake. The only thing I could think of that qualified me for the position was that I had not sought it; in fact, this calling was the very last thing in the world I would have asked for.

Janet put the calling into perspective for us, as is her tendency, by comparing the commitment we were making to the paying of tithing. Sometimes, she pointed out, some of us could conclude that with all our financial obligations, there is no way we can give the Lord 10 percent; but if we do, there will always be enough. So I concluded that while it appeared I had no time, I would find a way to give the Lord what little he was asking for.

At about the time I was called, our fourth child, Michael, developed acute appendicitis, which required surgery. But I immediately found that serving as bishop helped me keep my own small problems in perspective, and I was able to view my concerns as nothing more than passing inconveniences. The calling also helped me focus more of my energy on my family and my friendship with Janet, knowing as I did that if our relationship remained strong, everything else in my life had a way of falling into place.

Janet: By November 1986, our daughter Wendy was engaged, and our son Tom's relationship with Kimberly was getting serious. On Thanksgiving and Christmas, our house was filled with family and friends. Rex and I couldn't help but rejoice in the four-generation span, from our parents down to our granddaughter. These were the first holidays we had all shared together in years, and they were delightful. Unfortunately, on

December 28 my sister's daughter Amy called to tell me that her father had left home. This announcement came as a complete surprise and caused me to reflect on Lois's and my talk as we had walked along the beach two months earlier.

Not long after, I began to have thoughts similar to those I had shared with Diana some months before—premonitions that some challenge lay ahead for me. My prayers increasingly included the plea that my family and I would be strengthened and be able to handle whatever we might face. One day in March, as I was in my bedroom praying, I was overwhelmed with the feeling that my praying for strength had more meaning than my rote recitation suggested. I didn't like this feeling, which tied my stomach in a knot, so I quickly ended my prayer and started in on the daily laundry. Still feeling unsettled, I began sorting the clothes. But when I was unable to concentrate on even this simple task, I knew I needed to return to my bedroom and resume my prayer.

I promised the Lord that I would do whatever was required of me. Then I ended my long and fervent prayer with what I knew was a selfish request. I pled for a two-month postponement of whatever change was going to take place. I wanted with all my heart to peacefully enjoy the two upcoming weddings of our children, to be able to celebrate unhampered with challenges.

Rex: Being the thoughtful, sensitive husband that I am, I had no idea Janet was experiencing such feelings. My primary focus was on what were without question the busiest three months of my life. In addition to serving as bishop, playing a minor role in our children's wedding plans, and dealing with the separation of Janet's only sister from her husband, I was scheduled to argue five cases between February and April 1987—two before appellate courts and three before the Supreme Court.

As I moved toward the most hectic three weeks of these months, I learned the outcome of the three cases I had argued before the Supreme Court earlier in the term. The results could hardly have been worse, as we lost two of the three. But I knew that I would live to fight another day—and that those three outcomes could not affect my efforts in the cases left to be argued.

Besides, I knew that despite the Court's mistakes, I would find great joy in upcoming family events: within days I was going to become grandfather of a second grandchild, and soon after arguing my final case for the term, I would head home for Wendy's wedding on April 25. My life was hectic but happy.

Janet: Being married to Rex, I had learned that timing is everything, especially in regard to important family events. Five days after Rex argued his final case of that term, we sat in the Salt Lake Temple as our daughter Wendy was married to Tom Jacobson.

The simple sacredness of the ceremony touched me deeply, and as I gazed at our beautiful children dressed in white, gratitude for their goodness prompted predictable mother's tears. I again felt as I had at Diana's wedding. I also recognized that our family ties would gain increasing significance as our family circle continued to grow. Through Wendy's marriage we had gained a new son, and when our son Tom was married in a few short weeks, we would be adding a delightful new daughter to our family. How wonderful they all were. I marveled at their righteousness and my good fortune.

We hosted a reception in our home that evening, complete with apple blossoms on the trees lining our driveway. Late that evening, after we had said goodbye to the newlyweds and the last of our guests, Rex and I looked at our kitchen—and at the task of restoring order to the entire house.

As busy as Rex has always been professionally, he often helps when there is work to be done, especially after big events. So I was more than a little surprised when, after we had surveyed the damage, he apologized for being so tired and asked if I would excuse him so he could get into bed. I reminded myself that given all he had been doing, his exhaustion was understandable, but I was disturbed by his out-of-character request. I knew that if he didn't have enough energy to help me, his fatigue must be extraordinary.

The next week, we all gathered in Virginia for an open house hosted by Tom Jacobson's parents. As is usually the case, the trip included meetings Rex had scheduled with his law firm, so we arrived a few days early and I had some free time. One morning as I drove to McLean to visit friends, my earlier feelings of concern returned with a vengeance, and I somehow realized that my challenge would involve Rex. This sense of foreboding was strong, and I was frightened.

I had absolutely no idea what that challenge would be, but on that warm, still evening in May, as the two of us drove along the George Washington Parkway to meet friends for dinner, I poured out my heart to Rex, although I said nothing specific about the impressions I had received. I told him how perfect our life was, how much I loved him, and how much I appreciated the years we had shared. Then, as my eyes filled with tears, I told him that I knew life wouldn't always be this perfect and that I wanted him to know our life together had nevertheless been everything I had ever wanted or dared dream of.

Not knowing quite what to make of all this, Rex tried to soothe my emotions as we drove along the parkway. It was obvious that he was a little perplexed by my outpouring.

The next morning, Rex and I drove to a familiar jogging path and ran along the banks of the Potomac River as we had so many other Saturday mornings. We talked and laughed like children, and even though we were in Virginia to celebrate the marriage of our third child, we were filled with a sense of youth—and invincibility.

After reminiscing about our Washington years, which had ended only ten months earlier with our move back to Provo, we talked about each of our seven children and the richness of our family life. I suddenly felt a bit somber as we neared our starting point, and I said to Rex, "What if something happened to one of us—an accident or illness—and we couldn't run together? I wonder what it would feel like to have one of us go off on a morning run while the other had to stay at home."

Rex, never fond of the hypothetical, listened and then gave me both a boyish grin and his answer: "Oh, I would tell you all about the run when I got home, and you could share the fun vicariously."

Then he added, "I'll race you to the car," and, having given himself a head start, he of course won.

That would be our last run together for well over a year.

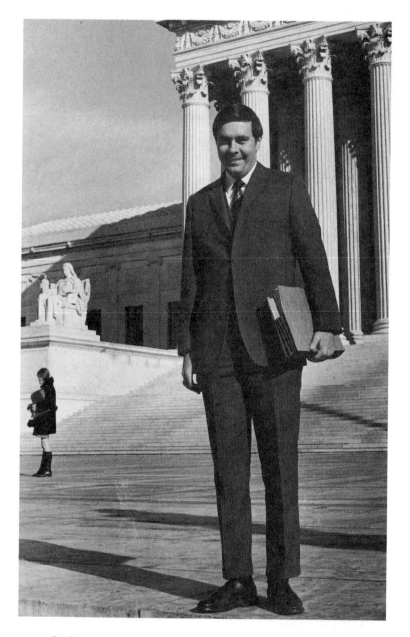

REX'S PRACTICE BEFORE THE UNITED STATES SUPREME COURT,
WHICH BEGAN IN THE 1960S, ULTIMATELY LED TO HIS ARGUING
FIFTY-NINE CASES BEFORE THAT COURT.

CHAPTER 2

"Can I Cry Now?"

Rex: In mid-May, as I reflected back on Wendy's wedding and looked ahead to Tom's, I saw myself living as interesting and fulfilling a life as anyone could hope for. Between being Janet's husband, sharing with her our seven wonderful children, serving as bishop, practicing law, and teaching at BYU, I could not imagine any combination of activities that could have made me any happier.

Tom, Michael, and I had just gone on our last fathers and sons' outing together before Tom's wedding. We enjoyed an outstanding meal together Friday evening—steak, onions and potatoes cooked in a dutch oven. (We fancied ourselves great cooks, but the deliciousness of the meal was actually attributable to two things—Janet's choices at the grocery store, and our dire hunger.) On Saturday we shared the adventure of wild water as we rafted on the Green River. A week later, I spent an evening in Washington, D.C., with Wendy and her husband, Tom, who had been married for just over a month and who demonstrated during our visit the early signs of a great life together. (His only real problem is that his first name causes no end of confusion at family gatherings.)

During the last week of May, I traveled to Oregon to speak at the commencement exercises of the Lewis and Clark Northwestern School of Law. While I was there, a good friend who practiced law in Portland asked if I would like to go running with an appellate specialist in his firm who was also an outstanding long-distance runner. This was a winning combination in my mind, so off the two of us went one morning. We were running up and down some pretty good hills, and before long I was huffing and puffing as if this were my first time running. Frankly, I was a little embarrassed; after all, we have much steeper hills in Provo, which is a good four thousand feet higher than Portland. But I kept up as best I could, mystified by my lack of energy.

Partway through our run, we heard a moaning sound from the side of the road, so we stopped and discovered a wheelchair athlete who had gone off the road and couldn't get back up. My running partner and I made our way down a rather steep embankment and pulled this fellow and his wheelchair up the hill. As we continued on our run, I became aware of a pain in my back—which didn't particularly surprise me, given what we had just done.

That evening, I attended a reception for the law school graduates, and after about twenty minutes, I was just too tired to stand. So I asked for a chair and sat for the rest of the event, during which I began to wonder why I was experiencing this decrease in energy.

The next morning, I delivered the commencement address and then headed straight for the airport, where I found that I was facing a four-hour delay before my flight would leave for Salt Lake City. In general, nothing frustrates me quite as much as schedules that aren't met; but my lack of energy, which I figured was the result of some sort of virus, put me in a reflective mood. So I set my briefcase aside and thought about the significance of the day—May 30, 1987—the fiftieth anniversary of my parents' marriage.

My biological father had been killed in a hunting accident about four months before I was born, and just after I turned two my mother married Wilford Shumway, the only father I have ever known. He couldn't have been a better father. My parents' anniversary, which we would celebrate together the following week, brought to my mind how important families are, both temporally and eternally. As I thought about my parents' marriage, I projected ahead twenty-two years to Janet's and my fiftieth anniversary and wondered what life would be like for us at that point. I wondered if I would still be running and practicing law at the age of seventy-four, and I thought about each of our children, the youngest of whom would be thirty.

But mostly I thought about Janet. For the past several months, we had been watching her sister go through a painful separation that had taken us all by surprise, and Janet and I had watched several other couples we knew go through similar ordeals. Although I'm not certain a twenty-four-year-old ever knows all he should about picking the right eternal partner, I knew when I married Janet that I was making the right decision, and I had grown increasingly convinced of my youthful "wisdom" over the subsequent twenty-eight years.

I had also figured out early on in our marriage that I was happiest when Janet was happy. This reality had nothing to do with demands she placed upon me; rather, I had learned that in pursuing my professional interests, I could not afford to lose sight of my wife and our children. They were the most important part of my life. In my reflective mood, I realized that I needed to direct increased focus toward enriching our relationship, as Janet had always done.

As the time finally came for my flight to leave, I called my father and mother to wish them a happy anniversary and then decided I could forgive the airline for the delay—as long as Janet hadn't become completely frustrated while waiting for me on the other end.

After my trip to Portland, I continued to feel run-down and tired, which cut into my running and my ability to work as hard as I was used to. But I also found that this condition had a rather pleasant tranquilizing effect on me, and I received comments after a couple of speeches indicating that my slower, more deliberate manner was viewed by some as an improvement on my sometimes rather hurried manner of speaking.

As we neared Tom's wedding day, I was reaching the point of exhaustion, and my back was still bothering me. I described my fatigue to a physician in our ward, who said he thought I was probably just suffering from a virus, and my back pain was attributable to my experience in Portland.

At this point, the thought of cancer never really entered my mind, although it had some months earlier. For years I've had a soft spot on the back of my head, which has been diagnosed as a harmless subaceous cyst. But in February I had noticed a lump under my right arm. This was at such a busy time that I knew I couldn't afford to be sick or even take time off for tests, so I had rather informally asked about the lump and had been told that it was probably just another subaceous cyst. That was exactly the answer I wanted, so I did not pursue the matter any further.

Janet: A few days after Wendy's wedding, my mother had emergency open-heart surgery, followed by a mild stroke. I helped her as best I could in the midst of preparing for Tom and Kimberly's wedding. With all that was going on, I was not as aware as I should have been of Rex's fatigue. And while I knew his back was hurting, I attributed it to his experience in Portland. My suggestion was that if his back continued to bother him, he probably should have it checked—after the wedding and luncheon on Thursday, June 18, and the reception in Boise on Monday, June 22.

Rex and I attended the beautiful wedding ceremony in the

Salt Lake Temple. Once again my soul rejoiced as I witnessed the sacred marriage of another child. We had all loved Kimberly instantly. She was as perfect for Tom as Steve Allred and Tom Jacobson had been for Diana and Wendy. We hosted a wedding luncheon, at which Rex served as master of ceremonies as we welcomed and visited with Kimberly's family, our family, and other guests.

After the luncheon, my sister, Lois, asked me if Rex was all right. "He doesn't look well," she remarked, and I was momentarily alarmed at her comment. I felt Rex was a very young fifty-two. He had been energetic and healthy his whole life, and the thought of him being sick enough that someone would notice made me shudder.

I left early the next morning to take care of my mother, who was recovering in nearby Summit Park. As I drove through Provo Canyon on my way to my parents' home, I was concerned about Rex, but my experience told me that whatever he had would pass quickly and that he would soon be back to his normal, healthy self. Our newlyweds were on a brief honeymoon to Sun Valley, and Rex wanted to be feeling well by Monday, when we would attend their wedding reception in Boise.

Rex: I spent all day Friday working on a motion that needed to be filed in the United States Supreme Court, and by the end of the day I had faxed copies to the other lawyers working on the case, who were in Chicago, Washington, and Mississippi.

On Saturday, I spent the day at a ward outing in American Fork Canyon. Because I was the bishop, I wanted very much to set the example of having a good time, but it was apparent to the ward members that I was in pain, despite my best efforts to act otherwise. When asked, I reluctantly acknowledged that I was having some back trouble. One friend tried to relieve it by picking me up by the chest and bouncing me up and down in his arms. That didn't work. Another gave me an over-the-counter pain reliever. That didn't work either. Then one of the ward members, a physician, gave me a prescription muscle relaxant. That at least took some of the edge off the pain.

I appreciated all of the efforts people made to help me at the party, but I was especially touched by my son Michael, who showed a concern and compassion for me that I found quite remarkable. He had just turned sixteen a few weeks earlier, which placed him squarely on the frontier between childhood and adulthood. And that day he demonstrated the best traits of both: the love and worry of a child for his father, mingled with a grown-up willingness to assume responsibility for the care I needed so much. All day long, as the other teenagers engaged in activities that are attractive to the young, Michael joined with them. But I noticed that he never let me out of his sight, and he came over often to ask what he could do to help.

Of course, Michael was more than willing to drive us home late that afternoon. When we got home my pain was so intense that I could not walk without his assistance. Michael recognized the severity of the situation and began calling every doctor on our ward list. He had a hard time finding anyone home on a Saturday afternoon, but finally we reached Lyman Moody, who was just on his way to Salt Lake City. I told him the muscle relaxants had helped quite a bit but that I didn't want to take any more without his prescribing them. Lyman said he would phone in a stronger prescription, which Michael went to get.

With Janet at her mother's house, Michael did not want to leave my side, even though he had a date that night. I finally convinced him that the pain had sufficiently subsided and that it was all right for him to go. I then called Janet to let her know I wasn't doing very well. She returned home immediately, which made me feel guilty for having called: at that point I thought her mother really was sicker than I was.

I was a little worried about the pain, but against Janet's wishes, I went to church the next day, although the muscle relaxants made it difficult for me to stay awake during sacrament meeting. I did the best I could through my interviews after church and then went home to bed. That evening, Lyman came to our home, and after doing the usual thumping, listening, and poking around that doctors do, he told me that I needed to have some X rays taken of my back the next morning. I told him this presented a problem because we needed to leave very early for Tom and Kimberly's reception in Boise, so he scheduled the tests for 6:00 A.M.

On Monday morning, I drove myself to the Utah Valley Regional Medical Center, had the X rays taken, and waited as my friend Bruce McIff, a radiologist, analyzed the results. He pointed out that one of my vertebrae had diminished to about 40 percent of its normal size, and he immediately sent me for a CAT scan.

When I came out of that test, Lyman was talking on the phone to someone I assumed was another doctor, and I heard him make the statement I will never forget: "So they are definitely destructive lesions." When he received the confirmation, hung up the phone, and turned to face me, I asked him, before he had a chance to say anything, "Lyman, what are destructive lesions? Does this mean I have cancer?"

He responded, "Rex, I'm afraid it does."

There was simply no time to discuss my situation, and there were many more tests that would need to be done, so Lyman took me by the arm and walked with me to the hospital pharmacy, where he ordered for me two kinds of prescription pain pills. Then he walked me out to my car and told me to come back in the next day so they could run the tests needed to determine exactly what kind of cancer I had and how far advanced it was.

As I got into my car, I was acutely aware of my physical pain, but my mind had gone numb. The only thing I could think to do was to bow my head, close my eyes, and pray that Janet and I would both have the strength to endure whatever came—and more specifically that I could somehow get through the rest of that day without spoiling it for Tom, Kimberly, and the rest of my family.

Janet: On Sunday, three different doctors in our ward had commented to me about how sick Rex looked. His skin had taken on a sickly pallor, and I could no longer deny that there was something very wrong with him. But I could not have been prepared for what I was about to hear when the phone rang early Monday morning as we were packing to leave for our trip to Boise. It was Lyman, who wanted to tell me before Rex got home that he had cancer. He had spoken to me a few minutes earlier in vague, elusive terms, but he was calling again to let me know what Rex already knew.

In a state of shock, I managed to ask Lyman whether we should go to Boise or not. His response was simply, "Go, and take your family pictures. I really don't know what is ahead for you and Rex."

As I hung up the phone and tears welled up in my eyes, Rex walked in. We looked at each other, and he asked, "Do you know?" I answered yes, and we embraced. Before we could say another word, the room filled with children waiting to leave for Boise.

A friend in our ward, knowing of our trip and of Rex's severe back pains, had offered the use of his van so that Rex could lie down on a bed in the back of the van during the six-hour trip to Boise. We got Rex situated and as comfortable as possible, the children climbed in, I got into the driver's seat, and we headed off for a 7:00 P.M. reception.

We thought the children had no idea what was wrong with their father. We later found out that our youngest child, Christie, had heard my conversation with Lyman and had informed the others that "Dad has cancer," having only a vague idea of what that meant. Christie was prone to occasional overstatement and misconstrued facts, and her siblings viewed her as less than credible. But while no one wanted to believe Christie, their father's pain could not be concealed.

My first thoughts were that my husband was going to die. He had scarcely been sick in his life, but I surmised from what Lyman had said that Rex would not live for more than a few months. I thought of our two children who had just been married and contemplated the likelihood that their children would never know their grandfather. I rather irrationally concluded that they would not want to come to our house because I would be a widow, and I imagined they would want to spend their time in a home with both a grandma and grandpa. I realized that our granddaughter Ashley, who was only three, would have only the faintest recollection—if even that—of a grandfather who absolutely adored her, and that her baby sister, Chelsea, would not remember him at all. As my thoughts painted all these pictures of life without Rex, my mind began to go numb—as a shield, I suppose, against emotions I didn't know how to handle, particularly in light of what we had to get through that day.

Our daughter Wendy, who had come from Washington, D.C., for her brother's wedding, was sitting in the front of the van with me. After half an hour or so, she asked, "Are you okay?" I instinctively said yes, but then, knowing that I wasn't fooling her, I corrected my "yes" with a whispered "no." Although I gave no explanation as to what was wrong, Wendy volunteered to drive so that I could get in the back with Rex.

By this time, the tension in the car had eased a bit, and the children had started listening to music. I thought Rex and I could have a moment together to share our feelings about the terror we were both feeling inside. So as Wendy took over the driving, I climbed into the back. Rex was working on pages of figures he had been writing on a yellow legal pad, however, and instead of the tender moment I had anticipated, he said, "Okay, I want to go over our financial situation with you. This is what we've got in the bank, this is what little insurance we have, and this is what I think you can live on."

That was not what I wanted to hear. I wanted everything to stop. I wanted the car to stop, the day to stop, and Rex to stop talking that way. I had just been given the news that my husband had cancer and that the outlook was bleak, and instead of our sharing the feelings we had for each other or our fears of what was ahead, he was calculating our finances. I stared at the yellow pad, but the figures blurred. My mind played tapes of our lives together and then went blank altogether when I tried to imagine life without Rex. The emptiness and fear that was gripping me had nothing to do with numbers on a piece of yellow paper.

Rex: Since I had left the hospital that morning, my thoughts had revolved around two basic themes. The first was that I had cancer, and to me that meant I was going to die. The second was an overwhelming concern for Janet and our children; my initial means of dealing with that was figuring out how they could get by with me gone. Frankly, I had not done a very good job of preparing us for such a possibility, and the financial reality looked quite bleak. (Years later Janet commented to me that her financial well-being was the absolute furthest thing from her mind as she climbed into the back of the van. I still maintain that it would have become a very real issue very fast if I had died.)

There were also two subthemes that kept running through my mind. The first was my desire not to spoil Tom and Kimberly's wedding reception and honeymoon, which meant I needed to put on a very brave face that evening, even though I could not imagine how I was going to stand in a receiving line for two or three hours. The second was my almost immediate recollection of my dear friend Terry Crapo, who five years earlier had died ten days after his cancer was diagnosed. He had been as close to a brother as anyone I had known (in fact, when we were attending BYU people often mistook us for each other), and I took his death as a very real indication of what was in store for me.

The reception that night was an ordeal—there is no other way to describe it. I did my best to be pleasant and effervescent—in other words, to act in a way that was completely foreign to my feelings at the moment—but I couldn't fake it completely, and I spent a good part of the evening sitting on a stool rather than standing. It was obvious to Tom that I was not feeling well, and several times he got out of the reception line to ask Janet if I was all right. She simply told him that I wasn't feeling well and that I was going to have some tests done when we returned to Provo (which was the truth—up to a point).

After the reception, Kimberly's parents invited us to their home to watch the happy couple open their presents. This was absolutely the last thing in the world I wanted to do, but in keeping with our effort to preserve the evening for Tom and Kimberly, we went.

While Janet and I were there, I received a call from our home teacher, Rodger Galland. I have no idea how he tracked us down, but he informed me that he would be at the Boise airport the next morning to fly us back to Provo and that he would bring someone to drive the van back. I protested, seeing no need for him to go to this trouble and expense, but Rodger simply responded, "You don't understand. I am going to be at the Boise airport in the morning, and then I'm flying back to Provo. If you and your family would like to be there, that's up to you." Seeing no point in Rodger's flying back to Provo in an empty plane, I acquiesced and thanked him for his thoughtfulness.

Janet: By the time we finished opening presents and headed back to our hotel, it was almost midnight. Five of our seven children were staying with us, and the original plan had been that two would stay in Rex's and my room and three would stay next door. Wendy sensed that we needed a room for ourselves and suggested to her younger brother and sisters that they all stay in one room and have a little party together. So finally, some fifteen hours after we had been told of Rex's condition, he and I were alone together.

As I shut the door to our hotel room, I turned to Rex and said, "Can I cry now?" He was in such excruciating physical pain that I don't think he had the strength to deal with either of our emotions, and he quietly said, "No, please don't. Just help me out of this tuxedo."

The painkillers Lyman had given Rex made it possible for him to sleep at least fitfully through some of the night, but I had no such luxury. In the darkness, I struggled to absorb the news of Rex's illness. Once or twice I dozed briefly, and each time I awoke, my first thought was that this was all a bad dream. Then I would see that I wasn't in my bed in Provo and realize that the news of Rex's cancer was an unalterable reality. I prayed off and on throughout the night for strength and for the relief of Rex's pain. I wished desperately for two things: that I could be the one with cancer so that Rex would not have to endure whatever was ahead, and that morning would finally come so that I could find some relief from the night.

Before the sun even slipped through the crack in the drapery, I had showered and dressed, finding some relief in the familiarity of mindless tasks. But as I brushed my teeth, I could not brush away the bitter taste in my mouth; and as I looked at myself in the mirror, I could see a change on my face and in my eyes. I had seen the last of the carefree mother of seven and was now staring at the face of one who was terrified at what was in store for her husband and family.

As I looked at this stranger's face in the mirror, I heard Rex stir and then moan in pain, and I rushed in to help him. I was immediately struck by the absurdity of this change in roles. Through my seven pregnancies, he had been the one to take care of me. He had been the one with unlimited energy, and I wondered if I had the strength to become his caretaker. But as he awoke that morning, I knew what I must do—that there was no other choice.

Rex: Janet helped me get up and ready for the day, and she then got the children ready for the flight back to Provo. I knew the flight home would be a bit unnerving for her because she has a mild fear of private planes. As we walked up to Rodger's plane, she said to me, "Aren't you just a little afraid to fly in these small planes?" My answer was simply, "Who cares?"

My response pretty well summed up my feelings at that moment. I thought I was going to die, and I had concluded the previous day that I would not live to see another Christmas, which was just under six months away.

We were back in Provo before noon, and Janet and I went directly to the hospital for more tests. In particular, Lyman wanted to have the tumor under my right arm removed so that he could have it biopsied, and he had asked a mutual friend, Mark Fullmer, to do that surgery. Mark was reluctant because he had just worked through a full day of surgeries and wanted to be fresh before he cut into me, but Lyman persuaded him, telling him that the tumor was small and would be easy to remove. I was also anxious to have it removed so that we could get on with what needed to be done, and I used the plea of my friendship with Mark, who finally gave in.

Well, the tumor was quite large, actually—about the size of an egg—and Mark cursed Lyman through the entire operation, all of which I heard because he had used a local anesthetic. But the doctors finally held in their hands the key to diagnosing exactly what kind of cancer I had and then determining a course of treatment.

Janet: My mind was still numb as we went to the hospital, and while there were many things I was uncertain of, the one thing I did know was that I wanted to be with Rex through all the tests and procedures. I wanted to be a support to him, but I also wanted to know what was going on in my husband's body, mind, and heart.

The doctors were very gracious about informing me concerning everything that was done that week, including the surgery to remove the tumor. And when our friend Steve Freestone went into the lab to perform the biopsy, he invited me in to watch. I think he knew that the more involved I was, the easier it would be for me to deal with Rex's cancer—and that I would be more frightened sitting in halls and waiting than I would be looking with him at slides of the tissue.

As he was slicing the tumor and preparing the slides, he said to me, "Let's hope this is a lymphoma, because chemotherapy is very effective in treating that form of cancer." Never once did he suggest, as he conducted the biopsy, the hope that

Rex didn't have cancer, nor did he leave me alone in silence to wring my hands and wonder while the doctors did their work. Rather, he took me step by step through the process of determining Rex's exact condition.

The final diagnosis was that Rex had a non-Hodgkins, T-cell immunoblastic lymphoma. The doctors had hoped they would find that the cancer was a B-cell lymphoma, which is not as serious as the T-cell form, but such was not the case. They also determined that this very fast-acting cancer was in its fourth and final stage and that even with Rex's depressed immune system (the result of his low white count), chemotherapy was the only option available to us.

As much as I wanted—and needed—to be with Rex during all of the initial testing, my good friend Margo Freestone, Steve's wife, came to the hospital on Wednesday to give me comfort and encourage me to leave for a while. I knew Rex would need something to rest in when he was home, so later that afternoon, after I had taken Rex home to rest, Margo and I went to look for a recliner that would be comfortable for him. I was not very good company, but Margo was helpful as I walked through the store in a daze.

The next day, Rex and I were alone in the house for a little while—he in the recliner and me on its arm—when we began to read together a letter we had received from our friend Richard Wilkins. Richard had been a student of Rex's and had later worked with him both in the solicitor general's office and then as a BYU law faculty colleague. Their relationship had initially been much like the relationship of a father and son and then like that of brothers. Richard's letter, which was most encouraging and on which we reflected frequently during the coming months, expressed some very deep sentiments about their friendship and also expressed his confidence in Rex's ability to battle this cancer. I am generally much quicker to express my emotions than is Rex, but at this moment, as we read Richard's letter together, tears flowed freely from both of us. I took my husband in my arms and said simply, "I had always wanted us to grow old together." Rex responded, "I did too."

For that brief moment, we set aside tests and treatments and shared in a very few words what we had each been feeling since Monday morning.

Rex: Most of my time from Tuesday through Thursday was taken up by blood tests, CT scans, a bone marrow biopsy, and other delightful experiences. During that time, I had quite a bit of time to think, and I began to realize two things. The first was that I might not die—that cancer was treatable and people did survive. Sometime during these days, I picked up the idea that I had about a 35 percent chance of recovering, and I decided that I might as well be one of that large number of individuals who made it. (Janet would later reinforce my view with a motto that came to have great meaning for us: "You are not a statistic.") The second realization was that there were three factors that were essential to my recovery: outstanding medical care, the faith and prayers of many people, and Janet.

Janet, I could tell immediately, would play a most important role in my recovery. She was with me constantly, providing support and encouragement, and she became an active part of the team that made decisions affecting my treatment and care.

Janet and I began the difficult task of explaining my illness to the children in terms they would understand. It was hard to convey to the youngest two how serious my condition was. Janet talked with Wendy and Diana by phone, and she discussed with Michael the medical terminology. Stephanie was on a school tour, and when Janet finally reached her by phone, she had just begun explaining the situation when an operator interrupted, saying their time was up. "This is an emergency and I'm talking to a child—please don't disconnect us," Janet said. "I'm sorry," the operator answered coldly. Then the phone went dead.

I spent a good part of Wednesday, June 24, telling my colleagues at the BYU law school and at Sidley & Austin the news of my cancer. Even with the return of my optimism, it was an ordeal to acknowledge to this wide circle of my associates that I might well be dying; the task of conveying the news of my cancer made this one of the lowest days in my life.

But the day began with my receiving a phone call that would convey perhaps the best news of my professional life. Three months earlier, in March, I had argued an important case before the Supreme Court, a case involving significant issues of religious freedom and employment law. I was stunned when one of the clerks of the Court called that morning to tell me that the outcome was 9–0 in our favor. I had thought we might win, but the last thing I expected was a clean sweep. Of course, the lows of that day were lower than the highs were high, but I was grateful for the lift to my spirits that this news brought.

Tom was the last of our children to learn of my condition. He and Kimberly had been on their honeymoon, and when they returned to Provo, Janet and I took them into our family room and explained to them the real source of my back pain.

Under most circumstances, Tom is very strong and not particularly emotional, but on this occasion his tears came quickly, and he ran upstairs to a bedroom. In about five minutes, he came back down, put his arms around me, and said, "Dad, I love you so much." These were essentially the same words each of our children had expressed upon learning of my condition. They were simple words, yet they meant everything in the world to me as I dealt with the week's events.

The first step in treating my cancer had been radiation therapy, which arrested the deterioration of my vertebra and provided significant relief from my back pain. The next step—chemotherapy—was scheduled to begin Friday morning.

The telephone rang as Janet and I headed out the door that morning. It was Ben Heineman, the managing partner of the Washington office of Sidley & Austin. Ben had become a close friend during the year I practiced out of that office. I am not one to be late for appointments, but I also felt I should take the call from my friend. Ben's wife, Chris, was the medical editor for the *Washington Post;* and he explained to me that the moment he

had learned of my cancer, he and Chris had begun canvassing
the country to determine the very best treatment available for T-
cell immunoblastic lymphoma. Ben explained to me that with
my particular circumstances—a depressed white count and cancer in its final stage—I needed the most experienced and skilled
medical help possible and that, in his judgment, the best place
for me was the National Cancer Institute, which is part of the
federal government's National Institutes of Health (NIH) in
Bethesda, Maryland.

I do not adjust well to sudden changes, and my initial reaction was that I wanted nothing to do with Ben's proposal. I had
planned out my life for the next several months, and that plan
involved staying in Provo with the support and companionship
of my family. In addition, I had every confidence in the doctors
and medical personnel at our local hospital, and I saw no need
to travel to the East Coast for treatment. But Ben is not inclined
to back down from a position once he is convinced he is right,
so for the next several minutes, he was the irresistible force to
my immovable object.

He explained to me that NIH, which is a research organization, was studying my type of cancer and that they had two pro-
tocols for my kind of lymphoma. He also explained that NIH
had the finest infectious-disease center in the country and that I
would need that support, given that chemotherapy suppresses a
person's immune system and that I was therefore at high risk for
infections, due to my low white count. Ben added that because
NIH is a research hospital, it was critical that I not receive
chemotherapy from another source, because if I did I would no
longer be eligible for its program.

Finally he said, "You can certainly wait a day or two before
you take your first chemotherapy treatment in Provo. So as a personal favor to me, do at least this much. Talk to a Dr. Longo at
the National Cancer Institute before you make your decision."

Largely because I saw no other way of getting this tenacious
lawyer off my back, I consented, and Janet and I called Dr.
Longo. The things he said made a lot of sense, particularly the

ability of NIH to provide extensive attention to my depressed immune system. For what Ben and Dr. Longo didn't know, but what Janet and I were painfully aware of, was that my dear friend Terry Crapo hadn't died of cancer. He had died from the pneumonia he had contracted while undergoing treatment for his leukemia.

By the time we finished our conversation with Dr. Longo, Janet and I had at least begun to accept the possibility that, for all its inconveniences, Ben's idea might be the best one. I pointed out to Janet that it would be quite difficult for me to be two thousand miles away without her and the children. She immediately responded that she would go with me. I really protested this notion, largely because I felt the children needed her far more than I did, but she told me there was no way she would let me undergo treatments without her there and that we could work out an arrangement for the children.

I could quickly see that Janet was tending to agree with Ben and Dr. Longo, and by the end of the day, after prayerful consideration, we had decided I would receive my treatments in Bethesda, Maryland. As I went to bed that night, I was deeply moved by the fact that our friends Ben and Chris would invest so much time and effort in my behalf—and I was very grateful for Ben's persistence.

Two days later, on Sunday, three significant events occurred. First, my parents had arrived on Saturday, and Sunday morning before church, my father gave me a special father's blessing. Having my father with me at this time meant a great deal to me, as did the optimistic tone of his blessing. That was immediately followed by an anointing and sealing, which was performed by my home teacher, Rodger Galland (who would succeed me as bishop two years later) and by my next-door neighbor and stake president, Merrill Bateman (who would succeed me as president of BYU eight and one-half years later).

The words in Merrill's sealing were direct, straightforward, and unequivocal. He told me without any qualification that this disease would not take my life at this time, and then he said, "The Lord yet has other things for you to do on this earth."

The final significant event of that Sunday was the sacrament meeting over which I presided. In a rather matter-of-fact manner, I informed the ward members of my disease, although most of them were already aware of the cancer. I explained that I would be taking my treatments at NIH over six five-week cycles and returning to Provo for about a month between each treatment. I then told the ward that President Bateman had graciously agreed not to release me and that he was allowing my counselors to take a larger role during my absences. During that sacrament meeting, I felt an outpouring of love and support from every one of our ward members, and the effect was comparable to the two blessings I had received that morning.

Janet: In Rex's mind, his talk may have been matter-of-fact, but for everyone there, it was heart-wrenching. Rex's mother was sitting next to me, and we were so emotional that neither of us could get through an entire hymn. Tears flowed from the congregation during his talk. It seemed to almost everyone there that this was Rex's good-bye to the ward and that he would not be coming back—at least not as bishop and possibly not at all.

In addition to Rex's family, my parents and sister had come to support us, and after sacrament meeting everyone came back to our house. I have no idea what we ate, but we did have a meal. Then we made our final plans before Rex and I left the next day for Maryland and the children left to spend several weeks in Arizona with Lois and Diana.

The next morning, Rex's friend Reese Hansen, who had been associate dean of the law school and Rex's counselor in the BYU Seventh Stake presidency, came to take us to the airport. As we backed out of the driveway on that bright June day, I remembered how beautiful the apple blossoms had been for Wendy's wedding just two months earlier. Now the trees were vivid green, and I wondered, as I looked at our home, what stage the trees would be in when we returned. My first thought was that they would be bare—and that the rest of my life would be bare as well, like trees in winter. What I knew for certain, even with the faith I was trying to sustain, was that life would never, ever be the same.

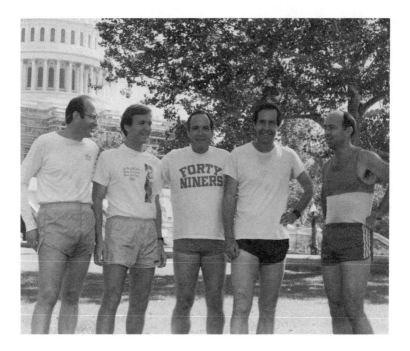

During his stay at NIH, Rex kept this photograph in his hospital room for motivation and inspiration. His running partners (l-r) are Cliff Fleming, Dee Benson, Stan Parrish, and Jim Croft.

CHAPTER 3

"Be of Good Cheer"

Janet: Rex slept during our flight to Washington, D.C., his system subdued as a result of the painkillers he was taking. I tried to sort out in my mind the events of the past week as well as to consider what was in store for us. When we arrived, we were greeted by Wendy and her husband, Tom, who were working in Washington that summer and would be returning to BYU in the fall. Wendy had been with us just a week before, during our trip to Tom's reception in Boise, but when she saw her father as we got off the plane, I could see in her face a sense of shock at his deteriorating condition.

Rex was so weak that we immediately got him into the car while we waited for the luggage. He asked for a drink of water, and Wendy volunteered to get him one; but when she finally got to the concession stand after waiting in a long line, she was told that they didn't sell water and couldn't give her a cup. She paid them the full price for a soft drink, told them to hold the ice and the soda, and filled the cup herself at the nearest water fountain.

Rex: While Wendy may have noticed a change in my physical condition and countenance, I noticed something in her countenance as well. As we greeted each other in the terminal, I did not see the slightest hint of shock. What I saw, instead, was a face filled with genuine care, compassion, and concern. Even more than that, however, I had the compelling impression that she wanted to do anything she could for me.

That moment at the airport typified something that would happen repeatedly as I was with my children off and on during these months. Even with the younger children—and certainly with the older ones—there was a maturity in how they interacted with and cared for me that brought joy to my heart each time we were together.

Janet: When Wendy finally returned with the drink of water, I was struck by how dependent on us Rex was—and sobered by thoughts of the challenges we were going to face in meeting even his most basic needs.

Fortunately, the staff at NIH was well equipped to help us, and it was something of a relief to bring Rex to a place where he would begin receiving the care he needed. During the first few days there, as tests were run and decisions about his treatment were made, Rex and I stayed in a nearby hotel although we spent nearly all our time at the hospital. Our intention was to find an apartment where we could both stay while Rex received his treatments, which we thought would give us some semblance of a life together, even with everything that would be going on at the hospital.

Rex: The treatment plan we had discussed with the doctors before coming to NIH involved six five-week cycles of chemotherapy, with a four-week break between each of the cycles. Although being away from my children, our ward, and our friends for five weeks at a time did not appeal to me, I consoled myself with the idea that Janet and I could live together in a nearby apartment, which my law firm had graciously offered to pay for; that we could return to Provo after each cycle; and that because NIH is a research institution, I would be paid for being one of their guinea pigs—in the amount of twenty dollars per day. Aside from the cancer, life did not seem all that bad to me. (Some, I should mention, have assumed that I was able to receive treatment at NIH because of my work in the government. That was not the case. The only qualification I had to meet to be admitted was to be suffering from a form of cancer the NIH research teams were studying.)

Our plans changed on the Friday after our arrival, when the doctors became concerned that the incision from which the tumor had been removed the previous Tuesday was infected. The NIH surgeons reopened it, cleaned it out, and decided that due to my depressed immune system, I would have to be treated on an inpatient basis for the duration of my chemotherapy. That Friday—July 3, 1987—marked the beginning of a four-month stay at NIH until the end of October. Even in my weakened condition, I had really been looking forward to spending the Fourth of July weekend with Janet, Wendy and Tom, and Stephanie. (We had rerouted Stephanie through Washington, D.C., on the way home from her school trip so we could see her before she went on to Arizona to be with her brothers and sisters.) It struck me as ironic that as the country was preparing to celebrate its independence, I was giving up mine.

When Janet left my room after I was admitted, Tom Jacobson noticed she was crying and attempted to comfort her. She thanked him but explained, "I'm not crying because I'm sad; I'm crying because I'm relieved that he'll now receive the care he needs." Her comment to him, I think, was indicative of both her insight and the seriousness of my condition.

On the one hand, being at NIH was very depressing for me.

Physically, it is a huge, stark facility; and even by hospital standards, it is a less-than-cheery environment. My room was very small, I could not move more than three or four feet away from my IV pole, and even though the hospital is situated in a beautiful part of Maryland, the view out my window was of another brick wall. Psychologically, I did not find it particularly uplifting that I was in an oncological ward that treats some of the most severe cancer cases in the country. I knew that many of the people in the rooms around me were dying, and even though I had recently felt renewed optimism and determination, the fact that I was surrounded by terminal illness weighed heavily upon me.

On the other hand, I was being treated by the most competent corps of nurses and doctors imaginable. Not only were they involved in cutting-edge research and treatments, which meant they had to be extremely competent professionally to be employed there; they were also concerned with me as a person. They were sensitive, compassionate, and easy to talk to, and they were willing to help Janet and me understand what we were going through. I knew that I had a good chance of recovering at NIH, and I was determined, as my status was changed from outpatient to inpatient that first day, that I was going to endure whatever it took to get better.

The plan on Friday was that if my infection cleared up, the chemotherapy would start on Monday. Frankly, if I was going to be stuck in the hospital over the weekend, I wanted to start that day. In my mind, there just was no point in waiting to begin the process of eradicating this deadly disease.

Janet: As we talked with the doctors at NIH about the procedures and possibilities in Rex's treatment, one of the first things we were told was, "Attitude is everything." And Rex's attitude couldn't have been better. After he was admitted, one of his nurses walked into the room, introduced herself, and said, "So, Mr. Lee, how are you doing today?" Rex immediately answered, "Well, aside from the fact that I've got cancer, I'm doing just great."

"We've got a live wire in there," the nurse reported as she pointed to Rex's room—and this was a pretty fair summation of his initial reaction to being at NIH. This was his chance to get better, so he was going to do exactly what the doctors told him and be the best patient he could be.

I, on the other hand, was still numb. From the moment I had learned of Rex's cancer, time had seemed to stand still, leaving me to go through the motions of life in an almost out-of-body state. I could barely eat, and sleep came fitfully in brief segments of the night when my exhaustion overcame my fear.

But that numbness gave way to reality as I pushed my husband in a wheelchair through the mazelike halls of NIH, going from room to room, test to test, and treatment to treatment. The first time I took Rex to the radiology treatment room, I encountered a woman who was pushing her husband in his wheelchair. They appeared to be in their late sixties, and he was so weak that he was bent over with his head nearly touching his knees. This very kind woman asked me what Rex's diagnosis was, and when I told her, she said, "Oh, I feel for you. We've been going through this for ten years now, and it's a lot to handle."

My first thought was elation that I might still have Rex with me in ten years. Then, as I looked down at my sick husband, I didn't know how I was going to find the strength I needed to deal with this unwelcomed intrusion in our lives.

On Saturday, several friends were getting together for a Fourth of July picnic. They prevailed upon me to go, even though I did not want to leave Rex alone. The picnic was held in a green meadow near McLean, Virginia, and everyone had brought their favorite food. At any other time, I would have enjoyed the visit with old friends, but that day I found it unnerving to listen to people laughing and having a good time. I just couldn't bring myself to join in the fun.

I also found it difficult to hear any of the less-than-kind words that are common to most couples. That evening such minor exchanges screamed at me in deafening decibels. I wanted to tell my friends that life is too short and precious—and certainly too fragile—to waste any of our time on petty differences.

Feeling more alone than I had ever felt before, I wandered away from the picnic tables, people, and party food and tried to find a place of solitude. I followed a tiny dirt road that seemed to lead nowhere in particular. As I walked, I longed to go home, to go back to a place I knew I could never be again—where there were no hospitals, no cancer, no fear of losing Rex.

Then, as I continued down the little road and saw the sun hanging heavy in the western sky, I began to feel the dirt and rocks through my sandals and I thought of the night that would soon come. Anticipating the loneliness I knew this darkness would bring, my mind turned to another who had walked the earth in sandaled feet, and I began to feel ashamed about feeling so alone. Then, as I recalled the Savior's promise to always be with us, I sat down on an old stump and contemplated that while the sun would set, it would also rise again—that there is an unerring dependability in these sequences of nature.

And then it occurred to me. My life was not out of control. The same God who set in motion the rising and the setting sun controls the universe, of which I am a part. And he had granted me my agency. So while I was faced with circumstances I did not understand and could not will away, I still had the ability to make choices in my life. The agency was mine, even if my ability to exercise it was limited to simply controlling my reaction to the events I was facing. No one, I knew, could take that away from me, and I prayed silently for strength.

As I walked back to the grassy clearing where the picnic was coming to an end, I knew there were sources of strength I had yet to find, and I also knew where they could be found.

That evening Wendy and Tom insisted that I come spend the night with them—and that I sleep in their bed while they took the couch. I found it slightly ironic that Wendy, for whom I had cared for since birth, and Tom, whom I had known since he was eleven years old, were now watching out for me. I accepted their kind offer, and for the first time in ten days I slept through the night. When I awoke the next morning, I began to feel that the numbness I had been experiencing was lifting a little, and I hoped that the Sabbath would bring relief to my aching soul.

When I attended fast and testimony meeting that day in our former ward, I shared my testimony and the news of Rex's illness. Many of the people there already knew and had joined together in a fast for Rex, as had our ward in Provo, the stake where Rex had grown up in St. Johns, Arizona, and, we later learned, other congregations around the country where we had friends and family.

After church, I went immediately to the hospital to see Rex. Before I went inside, I felt that I needed some time alone to pray. I went into a wooded area across the street from NIH and began, once again, to plead with my Heavenly Father in Rex's behalf.

I have known the fundamental elements of prayer from the time I was two or three. I prayed in my childhood, as so many children do, thanking Heavenly Father for my blessings and telling him what I felt I needed. As I grew older, I felt that my prayers had matured, and I learned to pray with a heart more open to God's will and to the guidance I know he gives his children.

For some reason, however, as I faced the frightening ordeal of Rex's cancer, I had forgotten much of what I had learned as an adult and had become a child again. In the first few days after the diagnosis, I must have sounded like a two-year-old, demanding and insisting that I have my way. "Please, Heavenly Father," I had begged over and over, "make him well." I had to pray. I knew nothing else to do. But these prayers did nothing to bring the healing balm I needed for my wounded spirit.

Soon, without even realizing it, I changed my prayers. I began to instruct, reason, even bargain with the Lord. "Surely," I would plead, "there are things on this earth for him to do. He is still useful here. Send him anywhere, ask him to do anything, and I will be at his side helping. Take away everything we own, but please leave him here." Again, I found no peace.

That Sunday as I bowed my head, my prayer was significantly different from my previous pleadings. "If it be thy will," I began, "let Rex recover from his cancer. Thou knowest the desires of my heart, but I recognize that I do not understand all things. Please strengthen me to meet the challenges ahead, and please calm my troubled heart." Finally peace came.

As I continued in prayer, I realized spiritually something I suppose I had known rationally—that changing circumstances isn't always an option, but that I could receive the strength I needed to deal with what Rex and I were facing. Scriptures I had known and loved for years came to my mind with new meaning. "Be of good cheer," I remembered from the Doctrine and Covenants, "for I am in your midst, and I have not forsaken you" (D&C 61:36).

Until that day, I had thought that faith in God came in the form of feeling certain that life would be as I wanted it to be. Coupled with that assumption was my fundamental outlook that I could find something good in whatever situation I faced. Now for the first time that premise didn't work. I could not see any element of good in the fact that my husband lay near death in a hospital bed across the street. But what I could see, as I concluded my prayer, was that my Heavenly Father was with me and would give me the strength I needed to get through this challenge.

The assurance that came to me that day was not that Rex's cancer would be cured forever, but that a loving and all-knowing God would be by my side. As I quietly arose to return to the hospital, I remembered the sentiment expressed somewhere in a biography of C. S. Lewis—that we do not pray to change God; we pray to change ourselves.

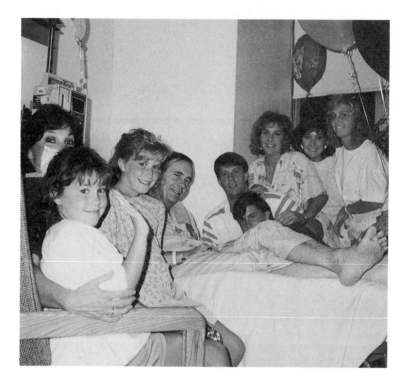

In August 1987, while Rex was a patient at the National Institutes of Health, Rex and Janet's seven children came for a week-long visit. Left to right: Christie, Janet, Melissa, Rex, Tom, Michael, Diana, Wendy, and Stephanie.

CHAPTER 4

Sustained by Faith and Prayer

Rex: For fifty-two years, I had enjoyed nearly perfect health. I had been in the hospital only once, for a very short time, and would have much preferred the doctors' original plan of administering my chemotherapy on an outpatient basis. There was an immediate sameness about the food and routines that made me long for the freedom I would have had outside of the hospital. At the same time, I knew I had to maintain the perspective that my primary and really *only* objective was to get better. I concluded right away that if my getting better meant staying at NIH for several months, then that's what I would do—like it or not.

One of my first concerns was that the members of our ward deserved leadership from one who had the mantle of bishop, and because it was now clear that I would not be dividing my time between Maryland and Provo, I felt honor-bound to offer our stake president, Merrill Bateman, the option of releasing me. His answer was characteristically direct: "We're not changing bishops. You just concentrate on getting better."

Waiting from Friday until Monday, when the first chemotherapy was scheduled, was difficult. The radiation therapy that had been started in Provo was reintroduced at NIH on Friday, and it helped to relieve the pain in my back. I wanted to get going with the rest of the treatment plan, patience not exactly being my strong suit.

There were just too many things I wanted to do, and I didn't want to spend a day longer in the hospital than was necessary. I wanted to see Michael, Stephanie, Melissa, and Christie marry and graduate from college, and I wanted to see many more grandchildren come into our family. I wanted to see Tom go to law school and then be the one to move his admission to the Supreme Court. I wanted to see Michael go on his mission, and I wanted to complete my tenure as bishop. I wanted to see all of our children, together with their husbands and wives, get a good start on life.

But most of all, I wanted to grow old with Janet. I wanted the experience of sharing with my sweetheart the later phases of life, just as we had shared the earlier ones. As I lay in my hospital bed over that weekend, waiting for Monday to come, I spent considerable time thinking about how Janet had been the perfect wife for me during our twenty-eight years together. Her insistence on being with me at NIH was only the most recent manifestation of her commitment to our marriage—and to me.

Janet: My thoughts as we waited for Monday to come were considerably different from Rex's. His principal oncologist had described to us what Rex's intense chemotherapy would mean when he said, "What we are doing is killing both good and bad cells. Then we hope that the good cells will restore themselves and the cancer cells will not return. It's barbaric, but this is the only way we presently know of to destroy cancer cells."

When Monday came, Rex was so tired and in so much pain that he had to be taken for tests throughout the hospital on a gurney, and even then he was miserable. The thought of the nurses' putting what amounted to poison into my husband's veins was horrifying to me, and as we waited in the afternoon for the person to come in and administer the first dose, I was filled with anxiety. Rex in a sense, shared my anxiety, but his was the result of wishing the nurse would hurry and get there and start him on the chemotherapy so he could begin the process of getting better.

Rex: Before the chemotherapy was injected, I was told that this particular drug—the first in a five-drug cycle—could irritate the veins and therefore make it hard to administer. I had no difficulty at all tolerating it; in fact, about an hour after my first treatment, the extreme fatigue I had been experiencing began to lift, and I asked Janet for a yellow pad so that I could do some writing. This was the best I had felt in two and a half weeks, and I began to speculate as to the reason.

My first thought was that the chemotherapy was working wonders, but then Janet reminded me of the fact that literally thousands of people—from friends and family to total strangers—had been fasting for me the day before. But the timing was not right, I told her; the fast had occurred on Sunday and my feeling of almost sudden recovery was occurring on Monday. She then explained that these people weren't fasting that I wouldn't have cancer; that was already a given. Rather, they were fasting that the medical treatments I was to receive at NIH would be successful. The earliest those prayers could have been answered, she continued, was when the first chemotherapy was administered.

I began to cry as I contemplated the faith and prayers of so many in my behalf. I felt a mixture of gratitude for the efforts of friends and family and embarrassment that I hadn't immediately recognized the real reason for my rapid improvement. My renewed energy made me very emotional, very humble, and very grateful—both to my Heavenly Father and to so many people who cared about me. This was the first of many times during my four-month stay that I became aware of the effect of others' faith on my well-being.

I am accustomed to and appreciative of the Latter-day Saint practice of fasting in behalf of someone who is ill. But this concept was somewhat foreign to some of my non-LDS friends, including a colleague at the BYU law school, Jean Burns. Jean expressed her concern for me—often with a healthy dose of her wit—many times while I was at NIH. Her first note came days after the fast Sunday in July and said, in effect: "What's this business about a fast? In the first place, I don't understand how the word *fast* describes not eating. But even more mysterious is how my not eating can possibly cure your cancer. But on the off chance that you Mormons might have this one right, I want you to know that I'm doing my part and that during the entire month of July I will not eat any broccoli. Let me know if it works."

While Jean—probably purposely—misunderstood the fundamentals of the Latter-day Saint fast, her love and good humor (and, I believe, her faith) were an efficacious offering in my behalf as well.

Janet: When Rex asked me for a legal pad just after the first dose of chemotherapy was administered, I was somewhat startled—both because he had been so weak earlier that day and because this was not how I had anticipated us spending our time together in the hospital. When he was admitted to NIH, I imagined that I would sit at the side of his bed each day as we held hands, gazed into each other's eyes, and expressed our love for each other. And while we did share several such tender moments, I could also tell quite quickly that my scenario wasn't going to be what would sustain Rex through this ordeal.

With what little strength he had, Rex wanted to work. I was concerned that if he did, he wouldn't get the rest he needed, but a doctor finally explained to me that stress manifests itself differently in different people and that Rex was probably the type who would find resting in bed as unrelaxing and stressful as anything he could do.

Initially, I had a hard time accepting the idea that working would be beneficial for Rex, but an experience during our first week at NIH helped me see that he was not a typical patient. A young and obviously bright psychologist came into Rex's room one morning, offering to teach him biofeedback—training the mind to focus on certain images as a way of taking one's mind off of pain, illness, anxiety, etc. Rex looked puzzled for a moment and then, with no suggestion of disrespect, remarked, "I'll let you know if I need your help."

What Rex knew, at least intuitively, was that he didn't need help concentrating on something other than his cancer. That came very naturally to him as he turned his attention to work. And even though he was confined to a hospital bed, Rex needed to feel that he was a part of ongoing life. He needed to be productive, even with the limits the cancer placed upon him. So I somewhat reluctantly helped him set up an office at NIH; and then, rather than staring fondly into his eyes, I read legal briefs out loud to him when he was too sick to read them himself.

Rex: Though it was far from a full-time undertaking, I did carry on a fairly decent practice of law from my hospital bed. The Sidley & Austin office with which I was principally affiliated was just a few miles from Bethesda, and almost every day a messenger would bring briefs, letters, and memos from lawyers in the office and take back tapes I had dictated, briefs I had edited, and so forth.

I worked on about twelve different cases while I was at NIH, including two that I took on while I was in the hospital (one was later filed with the Supreme Court and another with the United States Court of Appeals for the Second Circuit). After a few weeks, Janet brought some order to my somewhat chaotic stacks of materials by organizing each case in an accordion file, all of which were then stored in a corner of the room.

On most days, I was capable of working only three or four hours, but they were fairly productive hours. At first, it struck me as strange that Janet wanted to be with me all day at the hospital—and even more strange that she would be willing to read legal briefs to me and do whatever other boring things I needed. Then it finally occurred to me that this was really what she wanted to do, that she was concerned enough about me to spend virtually every waking minute of the day with me.

(When I later told the law faculty at BYU about our months at NIH and how Janet would sit by my bed reading legal briefs to me, my friend Cliff Fleming, who teaches tax law, commented, "Oh, yes, my wife and I have spent some of our most delightful moments reading to each other from the Federal Income Tax Code.")

In addition to the work I did on legal matters, I was also concerned during the first few weeks at NIH about a commitment I had made earlier that spring. On July 24, the St. Johns stake where I had grown up was going to celebrate its one hundredth anniversary, and I had been invited to be the keynote speaker. I regarded this invitation as one of the highest honors I had ever been given, and if there had been any way for me to leave my hospital bed and be there, I would have done so in a minute. Of course, I couldn't, so I did the next best thing. I persuaded the stake president to let me write the talk and then have my father deliver it. The only problem was that it took me until nearly the last minute to dictate the talk, I had no way to transcribe it in the hospital, and at the time there were no fax machines in St. Johns.

Fortunately, my good friend Bud Jones had come from Arizona to visit me, and he offered to take the tape back to his law office in Phoenix, have it transcribed, deliver it to St. Johns, and fax a copy to me. Then my father and I went over the manuscript on the telephone, making the last-minute editorial changes we felt were necessary.

I explained in the introduction that "if this speech turns out to be anything less than a total smashing success, I will conclude that it was not because of the quality of the prose, but simply because my father failed to read it with the conviction and passion that its content deserved." Later I was told that my father interjected, "I cannot rise above the script." I appreciated my father's help, and I was glad that I could have at least this long-distance connection with a community that had had such a profound effect on the way I have viewed and lived my life.

Janet: Rex is a very conscientious person, and he was determined to fulfill all the responsibilities he could. He also made a point of remembering those things wives hope their husbands won't forget. Tuesday, July 7, marked our anniversary, and as I sat in his room that morning, looking out his narrow window onto the wall of another wing, I couldn't help but think that this was an unusual way to celebrate the day we had been married twenty-eight years before. I had never even thought about a life without Rex; and that morning, as I tried to construct an image of what that life would look like, I could see only a brick wall.

Our circumstances afforded us more time than we had ever spent together on an anniversary, and as Rex and I talked off and on during the day, I felt an increasing sense of sweetness and peace. The culminating moment, however, came that evening as Tom and Wendy brought Chinese take-out food to Rex's room, together with a small, wrapped box, which Wendy slipped to Rex. "I think this is exactly what you specified," she said to her dad. Rex then gave the box to me, kissed me, and wished me a happy anniversary.

I was surprised that he had thought to ask Wendy to buy a gift for me and regretted that I had not left the hospital to get something for him (although he had always told me that the best gift I could give him was to save the money). I removed the bow and wrapping, with Rex watching me intently. When I opened the box to find a gold chain with a single, perfect pearl, I noticed his eyes filling with tears. "You remembered," I whispered, as I sat on his bed to hug him.

His gift to me that night was identical to a gift he had given me two months before our wedding, as I left Provo to visit my parents in Japan where my father was serving as treasury attaché. "Think of me while you're gone," he had said. "Have fun but miss me, and remember to drink your milk." (His last instruction was his typical way of never letting a moment get too sentimental.) I had worn that necklace for years, until one of our babies had pulled it off and it had then disappeared.

The two gifts were alike, but the years had given this second gesture far more meaning than the first. And as Rex held my hand for the rest of the evening, I knew that, like me, he never wanted to let go.

Rex: Almost literally from the first day, my treatments had their intended effect on the cancer. The radiation therapy, which had immediately helped to alleviate the pain caused by my disintegrating vertebra, brought permanent relief; and with each dose of chemotherapy, my tumors receded in size.

The bad news was that the drugs also had the feared effect on my immune system. With each cycle, the pattern was the same. After the first three or four days of receiving the chemotherapy, I would begin to develop fevers and nausea. I had rarely experienced nausea in my fifty-two years—and then only in very short spurts—but now I constantly felt right on the verge of vomiting. Eating, which had always been such a pleasure, became a real chore. Within the first week, I had lost twelve pounds—and the weight loss didn't stop there. My doctors kept telling me I needed to gain as much back as possible because proper nutrition was an essential part of the total treatment, but the thought of ingesting food was absolutely repugnant to me. My ability to eat was further complicated when I developed, about two months into my stay, a hiatal hernia, which in its most severe episodes prevented me from swallowing at all for up to an hour or more at a time.

Not coincidentally, the nausea consistently and quickly followed the second drug to be administered in my protocol—nitrogen mustard. Chemically, it contains many of the same ingredients as the mustard gas used as a lethal weapon in World War I. As Janet and I asked about the various drugs I was being given, the doctors explained that the origins of chemotherapy could be traced to the autopsies done on victims of the war, which revealed that many of them had no lymph nodes. Researchers hypothesized, correctly, that something like mustard gas might be used to treat lymphoma patients. As I lay in my bed at NIH, I sometimes felt a little like a victim of war.

The nausea turned my body inside out and made my life a total misery, but even that was a relatively minor inconvenience when compared with the infections. They were caused by the depression of my white count below 500 and created quite a dilemma both for Janet and me and for the doctors. If we didn't continue the chemotherapy, I would almost certainly die of cancer. If we did, however, there was the very real risk that I would die of infections.

When the fevers came, they were first treated by potent intravenous antibiotics, which brought them down for a time. Then other fevers would occur, against which antibiotics were ineffective. Blood tests revealed the reason: these latter fevers were caused not by bacterial infections but by fungal infections in the blood. These infections were one additional complication stemming from my depressed white count, and antibiotics were ineffective in combating them.

In 1987, there was only one real antidote for fungal infections—amphotericin B (which is still by far the most effective for severe cases such as mine). This yellow liquid, administered intravenously, is known among members of the medical profession as "ampho-terrible," and the first time I received it, I learned why.

As the nurse attached a container of what appeared to be

about a liter of this liquid to my IV lines, she told me the administration would take about an hour and a half and that I should let her know if I had any unusual side effects. I asked her what I might expect, and she said the most likely was chills. That certainly didn't scare me. I was a big boy and I'd had chills before. I figured I'd simply put on an extra blanket and tough it out.

I fell asleep soon after this stuff started dripping into my veins, and after about forty-five minutes, I woke up and felt a little cold. The chilly feeling rapidly increased, and I covered myself first with a sheet and then with a blanket—all to no avail. Rather quickly the chills progressed to a stage far beyond anything I had ever known, and within minutes I was shivering so violently that the bed was physically moving. At that point, I rang for a nurse.

As she put the demerol into my IV—while I was literally bouncing around on the bed—a doctor came in, sat by the side of my bed, put his hand on my shoulder, and said in a very calm, reassuring voice, "What is happening to you is, of course, frightening, but in no way life threatening. With the demerol being injected into your IV, your chills will be gone in a matter of seconds."

His calm, reassuring words, combined with his rather commanding presence, had a very soothing psychological effect on me, and within about ten seconds the chills went away immediately and completely.

A few days later, I was given amphotericin again, and this time I kept my finger on the call button and rang for the nurse the instant I began to feel a chill. And after that, the nurse simply administered the demerol before injecting what I now joined the medical community in calling ampho-terrible.

The prospect of my dying occurred to me frequently during my months at NIH, and I did ultimately come to reconcile myself to that possibility. I did not want to, of course, for at least two reasons. First, the thought of death scared me. I have absolute faith in the existence of God and a hereafter, but I was not at all comfortable with the prospect of leaving this mortal existence just yet. But my much stronger reason was my concern for Janet and our children. Eight-year-old Christie, our youngest, along with Melissa, Stephanie, and Michael, were still at home and, in my view, needed a father. None of our three married children had been married very long, and I felt I should be there for them as they moved through at least the early years of marriage. And I did not want to leave Janet alone at a relatively young age.

Each night when I would pray, the principal thing I would pray for was to live. There were many days and nights when that did not seem like much of a prospect, but when I would plead with the Lord for my life, I would inevitably hear the words of President Bateman's blessing—"The Lord yet has other things for you to do on this earth." And throughout my darkest days, when my body was so weak that I could barely move, and when I was wracked with fever and pain, those words would give me the confidence I needed, despite their seeming incongruence with my situation at the time.

Janet: During the first several days that Rex was in the hospital, there were very few positive signs. After the first two doses of chemotherapy, his white count was down to under 50 (which was a level unheard-of, even at NIH) and the infections had started. His health was on a downward course from mid-July through most of September, with minimal promising indicators along the way.

While Rex's inclination was to get the best doctors he could find and then let them treat him, my approach was to find out everything I could about his form of cancer and then be an active part of his care and treatment. The staff invited me to use the well-equipped NIH library, so when I wasn't with Rex, I studied everything I could about non-Hodgkins, T-cell immunoblastic lymphoma. Doing that enabled me to ask intelligent questions of the medical staff, and in time the doctors and nurses began to treat me as something of a colleague as we watched Rex and worked to make him well.

At the same time, I would sometimes become very frightened as I learned more about the severity of his cancer and as I studied the statistics that related to his chances of recovery. When I would finally leave him in the evening, I often would drive back to my little apartment contemplating a situation that seemed increasingly bleak.

On countless occasions, either as I was falling asleep or when I would wake up during the night, I would be overwhelmed with a sense of panic. My heart would pound wildly and I would experience a shortness of breath. I just couldn't face the thought of Rex dying, because without him, I could not see me. Our lives were just too inextricably intertwined. And yet, although Rex had been told in blessings that his time had not come, reality seemed to indicate otherwise.

Absorbed in all I seemed to be losing, I would sometimes feel a sensation that I was free-falling and desperate for something to grab onto, something strong enough to stop the fall.

What I would grab onto at these times when I could not shut out the doctors' diagnosis were my faith and my ability to pray. I offered many prayers in the middle of the night. They may have seemed repetitive to the Lord, but they gave me strength to move past the overwhelming fear I was facing. I realized more fully than ever before that changing the circumstances is not always an option, but being given the strength to deal with what we are facing is the greatest blessing of all. There were many instances when it was hard for me to hold onto my faith—especially as doctors would describe to me what appeared at times to be very grim prospects—but it was all that I had. I knew that if I let go of that faith, I would never break my fall.

Rex: The central figure in one of the most poignant examples of the power of faith to heal was neither of my race nor of my religion. Her name was Juildene Ford, and she is the only nurse I know who still wears the traditional highly starched white uniform and cap. And during the time I knew her, she was just as serious about her professionalism and her religious devotion as she was about her orthodox nurse's attire.

My most serious episode with infections occurred one night in the latter part of August, during the second cycle of chemotherapy. I have very little recollection of that awful night except that I felt terrible and that Ms. Ford seemed to be taking my temperature at unusually short intervals. Then I remember the great relief I felt when my fever broke and Ms. Ford, after having taken my temperature for the umpteenth time, said to me, "It's okay now, Mr. Lee. You're going to be all right."

It wasn't until sometime later that Janet told me the story of what happened that night. After Janet left the hospital, she continued to call back and check on my condition because she was worried about the severe infection I was battling. The news she got was not good, and as the night dragged on, it got worse.

But the final report from Ms. Ford that night was this: "He's all right now, Mrs. Lee. His fever has gone down; in fact, his temperature is almost normal. But let me tell you what happened. I knew that with that high a fever and in his condition, he could not last through the night. So I went next door to the nurses' station, bowed my head, and prayed, 'Lord, this is too good a man to let die. Make his fever go down, and let him live.' Then I went back and took his temperature again. It had started to subside, and it has continued to do so since then."

I don't know, and will not know in this life, just how these things work—and why it is that sometimes they work and sometimes they don't. But it just may be that Juildene Ford is one of several people who saved my life, with assistance, of course, from her Heavenly Father and mine.

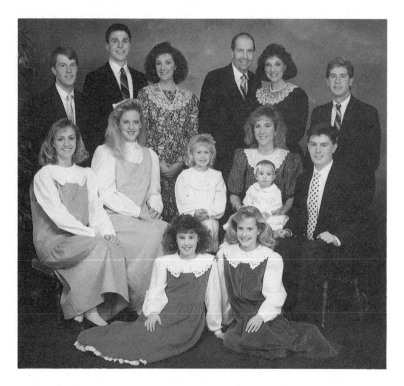

THIS FAMILY PORTRAIT WAS TAKEN AT CHRISTMASTIME 1987,
JUST AFTER REX'S STAY AT NIH.

CHAPTER 5

Happiness in Small Doses

Janet: It would have been much easier for me if life outside of Rex's hospital room could have ceased and I could have focused every last ounce of my attention on helping him get well. But there were still bills to pay, four children at home two thousand miles away to attend to, housing and transportation arrangements to make, and constant work to be done as we took care of the details of our changing lives.

I did many of my routine tasks while I was at the hospital with Rex. I figured family finances and balanced the checkbook while I sat by his bed, and there was a small room at the end of the hall with a toll-free telephone that NIH provided for the use of patients and their families. From there, I could keep tabs on our children and orchestrate whatever arrangements I could make from that distance to provide for their care.

We were fortunate that my sister, who was still living in Arizona, was able to take Michael, Stephanie, Melissa, and Christie from June through late August. Our oldest daughter, Diana, her husband, Steve, and their two children were living in Mesa, and they added to the large family circle for our temporarily "orphaned" children. Diana spent nearly every day with her younger siblings. Then in August, she brought the children back to Provo and helped them get ready for the new school year.

Diana stayed as long as was possible in Utah to help with our children, but her two daughters, Ashley and Chelsea, were only five months old and three years old, and she needed to get back to Arizona to be with Steve, who was beginning a two-year clerkship with a judge in Phoenix. Again we were able to find a solution to what seemed initially to be an insurmountable challenge. Wendy and her husband, Tom, were working in Washington for the first two months of Rex's stay at NIH; in fact, when Rex's status was changed to inpatient, they moved into my little apartment and provided great support to both of us through July and August.

Then, when it was time for them to return to Provo, they insisted that they could live in our house, keep up with their full-time schooling at BYU, and take care of Michael, Stephanie, and Melissa. Rex and I could not see how they could manage so much and argued with them to let us find some other alternative, but they would have it no other way. (In retrospect, we saw great blessings in the fact that during the years we lived in Virginia, Tom had been acquainted with the children he was to help care for.)

Starting in September we would send a check each month for their expenses. Tom initially tried to ration it out to ensure that they would get through the month. He was met with some resistance, however, and the typical pattern that evolved was that most of the money would be spent in the first two or three weeks. Then they would try to rein in their bad fiscal habits during the next little while, and finally they would spend the last few days of the month looking under sofa cushions for every last nickel they could find and praying someone from the ward would bring in a meal.

Emotionally, they fared much better than they did fiscally. I would call home most days with news of Rex's condition, and I admit that I tended to look for the best news I could to pass along. So while they knew their father was very, very sick, I tried not to scare them when things were particularly rough. Even so, it was hard for the children, but when one of them would get frightened, Wendy and Tom were there to help. We learned the extent of the efforts of this newly married couple when Melissa told me one day that she had been awakened by a nightmare the night before. I was worried about this, and I asked her what she had done to get over it. "Oh," she said, "I just went and got into bed with Wendy and Tom. That's what we do when we get scared at night, and they help us feel better."

Tom and Wendy dealt expertly with late-night homework assignments, procrastinated posters, and everything else children remember only when bedtime comes. It helped that Tom and Kimberly lived nearby and could assist with homework and join in weekend activities.

There was also the matter of taking care of myself. There were many people—doctors, nurses, friends in the area—who were much more concerned about me than I was. They felt I should leave the hospital more often, that it wasn't healthy for me to be there day and night. I knew full well that there is plenty to do in the Washington, D.C., area, and I was often told, "Get out and do something *you* like to do." I understood the concern my friends felt, even when that concern was unspoken, that I needed to redefine my own identity and see myself as separate from Rex. But the truth is, I was miserable anywhere I went without him. While their advice was no doubt right for some people (and through this experience I learned in many ways that what works for one person doesn't always work for another), I chose to stay with Rex as much each day as I possibly could.

As I did so, I found myself becoming an essential part of his care. I made good use of the library at NIH, where I could check out books that helped me understand his cancer, the chemotherapy, his nutritional needs, and the emotional side effects with which both of us would likely have to deal. I read books that explained each drug he was taking, with its origins, uses, side effects, and so on. I talked to every doctor and nurse who entered the room, made notes and lists of questions for the doctors, recorded Rex's various reactions to medications, and asked doctors about possible drug interactions. At times antibiotics adversely affected him, and I was glad my notes were helpful in identifying those reactions. I felt I was part of the team, I found relief as I understood his condition, and I personally benefited from spending more time on his care and comfort than on my own pursuits.

Rex made valiant efforts to work on cases and be productive, but much of the time he was just too sick or too tired to do so. I was always glad when he could sleep during the day and thereby find some relief from the agony his body was experiencing. There were several such moments when I was paying bills or doing something I needed to do, and I would glance at him while he rested. Sometimes he looked so peaceful and healthy that it was almost like a mirage, and I would think for just a second that when he awoke we would be able to leave this dreary place *together.*

My plan had always been that we would raise our children, go on trips, talk, read, run, walk, sleep, live—all of it together. Even with my own interests, his life was so much a part of mine that I couldn't seem to separate the two in my mind. I wanted to return to the life we had known, and I was filled with appreciation as he did everything he could to cooperate in the process of getting well. Rex has always shown a remarkable degree of determination—as a father and husband, as a lawyer, as a runner—and here he was, with so little strength, still showing that same determination. Even though I knew we weren't going to walk out of NIH together just yet, his efforts sustained me in my hope that one day we would.

Rex: In addition to all that Janet did in my behalf, which was a constant source of amazement to me, many other people provided me with support during my four months at NIH. Because of the risk of infection, I wasn't able to have too many visitors, and I was a long way from many who might have otherwise come to visit.

But I did receive many, many letters from friends—ranging from humorous get-well cards to short notes of concern to longer reflections on my condition. I had sometimes experienced the feeling of not quite knowing what to say when someone was sick, but I now saw how valuable such expressions of concern could be. I appreciated and was lifted by even the most simple expressions of love and concern. I also received many, many telephone calls, some from people who were Church leaders and government officials and who could have justifiably considered themselves too busy to take the time.

The nurses at NIH made a fuss over the fact that some well-known individuals called or visited—mostly, I think, because they knew the relationship between how a patient feels emotionally and how likely it is that he or she will eventually recover.

Once, just minutes after I received a dose of one of the chemotherapy drugs that always wiped me out, my nurse put through a call from Justice Harry A. Blackmun of the United States Supreme Court. Later she told me that as I spoke on the phone, she had said to herself, "This guy's a performer." I wouldn't have thought of my reaction in quite those terms, although I realized that my professional life did involve, in a sense, performing before Justice Blackmun and his associates. I probably did perk up a little when he called. But more to the point was that I was grateful to hear from a friend who cared about me. His concern lifted my spirits, as did the concern of so many others.

After I had been at NIH for about a month, I received a telephone call from our friend and very conscientious home teacher, Rodger Galland. During the conversation, he asked when we would be coming back to Provo, and I responded that it might not be until the end of the year and it would certainly not happen for several months. He responded simply that that was too long to be away from my children, and then we moved on to other subjects. The next thing I knew, some of our children called and said that Rodger had asked them to identify a time when his pilot and plane could take them all back to Washington to visit Janet and me. And that is exactly what happened. All seven of them came, including Diana, who was still living in Arizona. Rodger's instructions to his pilot were to stay there as long as our children could stay.

Janet: Even though I called our children often, long-distance mothering was no substitute for exchanging warm hugs, helping with homework, and providing reminders to practice the piano and clean their rooms. And as the summer passed, I could see that Rex's hospitalization was going to go on for several more months and that he was just too sick for me to even attempt a weekend trip home to see our children. So when our children told us of Rodger's offer, I had something to be excited about for the first time in weeks.

When our seven children walked into Rex's room, they were a beautiful sight, and Rex and I both burst into tears. Then we hugged, exchanged greetings, hugged again, and all cried together. Rex's small room had never held so many people, and the nurses came in to see this spectacle.

After taking pictures, asking and answering a host of questions, and talking about the good times we had shared and planned to share again, I left our son Tom with Rex and took the other children to settle into my small apartment. Our family has always thought that more meant merrier, and for the next five nights we confirmed the truth of that old adage—in rather cramped quarters.

The children seemed to have two goals in mind—to make me laugh and to make me eat. The first proved easier than the second as they tried to get my mind off Rex for at least a few minutes at a time. Somehow I felt strange the few times they took me away from the hospital, with Rex so sick, but I enjoyed our outings to the extent that I could.

Of course we spent most of our time with Rex, and I found it fascinating to watch each child with him over these six days. Diana, who has always known the workings of my heart, tried hard to cheer me up. She took almost a parental interest in my welfare, and when she realized I wasn't running she encouraged me by going with me. She brought pictures of our two little grandchildren and entertained us with those stories of extraordinary abilities that only grandparents want to hear.

Tom seemed to have matured in just the few weeks since Rex and I had seen him. His loving concern for his father was apparent as he stayed close to Rex's bed during most of their visit, and I could see that the thought of losing his father weighed heavily upon him. His relatively few weeks of marriage had also made him more tender and protective of my feelings as he reacted with newfound intuitions.

Then there was Wendy, who had been my constant support ever since our traumatic arrival at the Dulles International Airport in June. Only a few months earlier, her dominant preoccupation had been with bridesmaids' dresses and wedding reception arrangements. As her mother, I had helped her plan for the realization of her lifelong dreams; now, she focused on helping me deal with the disruption of mine. She was amazingly good at it, which was an interesting paradox that I saw in our other children as well. Almost overnight, she had grown in her perceptiveness and ability to comfort me. My situation was one I desperately would have willed away, but watching Wendy in this new role was the beginning of my awareness that good things can accompany adversity.

Michael was fascinated by the workings of the hospital and wanted to know every detail of Rex's treatment. His curiosity covered everything from the chemotherapy to the experimental laboratories at NIH, and I thought he was never going to leave the hospital, even to eat. His empathy for his father was tender and genuine, but his attitude was positive and enthusiastic. As I watched this sixteen-year-old, I missed the long talks and philosophical discussions the three of us had shared and hoped he would still be comfortable talking with us when Rex and I eventually returned.

I had tried hard to protect the younger children, especially, from worry, remembering how I had felt as a nine-year-old when my mother was taken away in an ambulance one day and then spent three months in the hospital, where she nearly died from asthma. I wondered if Stephanie realized the seriousness of Rex's illness, but I soon saw her concern for her father, which she manifested by keeping him entertained with her quick wit and her feigned knowledge of German, Italian, and French—complete with the appropriate accents. Underneath her fourteen-year-old self-assurance, however, we could see how vulnerable she really was. I wondered if she would be all right without us when she returned to Utah—and if I would be all right without her.

During her first day with us, Melissa, at eleven, would hug us one minute, get Rex drinks of water the next, and then run out the door to push Christie down the hospital halls in a wheelchair. (At one point, some thoughtful nurses came in with crayons and paper and invited our two youngest to use an empty room nearby to play in.) The next day, Melissa sat quietly on Rex's bed, asking about how he felt and whether he liked it at NIH. I worried that by the time Rex and I returned to Provo, Melissa would no longer be our little girl—that with the circumstances we were all facing, she would turn the corner into adulthood before she was ready.

Christie, our youngest, would climb onto her daddy's bed, snuggle for a moment, tell him he smelled like medicine, and then ask him how long it would be before all of his hair would be gone—and whether it would *ever* grow back. "I hope so," he told her, "but if it doesn't, I'll just take some of yours." She was full of quick questions that brought quick answers, and then she would join in wheelchair races with Melissa. She was about the age I was when I was separated from my mother for three months, and we decided that for her sake she would stay behind with Rex and me when the others flew home.

Later, her staying would prove to be as much for my benefit as for hers, as she always found some way to make me smile. Sometimes it was something funny she said; other times, as I would drive us home after visiting with Rex, she would literally reach over and turn up the corners of my mouth. Somehow she sensed that it was her responsibility to keep my life in balance and to make me smile, and during many dark days she did what no one else could.

As the days went by, I began to realize the circle a family makes as we love and take care of each other. These seven children had been our babies, whom we would care for always; but now, in Rex's and my time of need, they were taking care of us and helping to fill our sad hearts with joy.

We shared a wonderful week, much of it spent in Rex's hospital room, and when the children's plane took off, I cried harder than I had ever cried before, not knowing when we would see each other again—or exactly what the future would hold for our family.

Rex: Those four or five days with my children were a great lift to me during a very difficult time. I have joked both in private and in public about how home teachers could learn a lesson from Rodger about doing a little bit extra for their families. But what touched me more than planes and pilots was Rodger's thoughtfulness in my behalf. As I define friendship, the ultimate expression comes when someone else's welfare becomes as important as one's own. I felt this from Janet, from our children and from the many friends whose concern for my welfare and happiness approached the ideal taught by our Savior.

Janet: For the first two months that Rex was at NIH, I lived close enough to walk to the hospital each morning. Those twenty minutes often afforded me the one opportunity in the day for uninterrupted reflection. Obviously, I would spend much of that time thinking about our immediate needs and concerns, but I would also try to use the time to nourish my soul as well.

A recurring thought had to do with something I had heard many years before—that the most important word in the gospel is *remember.* I found myself linking this concept with a song I had begun singing as a very young child: "Count your many blessings; name them one by one." I remembered that my father often asked me, as he tucked me into bed at night, to tell him all the things I was grateful for that day, and he suggested that I remember these things in my prayers. I also recalled that when I was a teenager and didn't think life was fair, my mother would remind me of the words to this song. I remembered times from my youth when I would finish singing it and literally begin to count my blessings. I would never quite reach the end of the list, but in the process of counting, I would realize how much I had been given.

These seemingly simple lessons that I often remembered took on great meaning as I tried to look beyond the crisis we were facing and see, instead, the countless blessings that could still be found in Rex's and my life. I found great blessings in the smallest improvements in Rex's condition and smiled with sublime satisfaction when his fever dropped to 101 after having hovered at 104 for several days.

When Rex and I were first married, we would often say to each other, "I like us," which signaled to the other the great joy we felt in being together. Once, after I had held Rex's head most of the day while he vomited, I helped him brush his teeth, change his pajamas, and get back into bed. As he laid his bald, pale head on an equally white pillow, he turned to me and said, "I like us." That moment had as much meaning for me as any we had ever shared.

Maintaining a sense of gratitude in the midst of adversity was not easy for me to do but is necessary, I found, in order to crowd out the periodic feelings of frustration and discouragement that were an inevitable part of this trial. My sister and I wrote to each other regularly while Rex was at NIH and Lois was simultaneously going through her divorce. One particular line that we shared was "Life doesn't have to be perfect to be perfectly wonderful."

We were both learning that adversity does not erase all that is good and rewarding in life. Furthermore, we began to understand that we didn't need to try so hard in these trying times to make the whole of life wonderful. We were finding, instead, that we could be happy—even in brief snatches— despite the surrounding challenges.

My sister helped me learn an important lesson when she shared this thought in a letter: "I've come to acquire a testimony about adversity: its absolute necessity, its potential to help us grow, and, most of all, its ability to draw us closer to our Heavenly Father. I have a different understanding of adversity now, viewed not with despair or anguish or regret but with confidence that my loving Heavenly Father is earnestly trying to allow me to learn something very important—so important that he is actually willing to let me suffer in order to learn the lesson."

Coupled with the thoughts my sister shared with me was a letter Rex and I received from our longtime friend, Larry Wimmer. Rex and Larry had known each other since 1954, during their first years at BYU, and Larry's wife, Louise, and I had become close friends when we lived in the same apartment building while Rex and Larry were students at the University of Chicago. In the early 1980s, Louise had battled cancer herself. The cancer had gone into remission, but then, after it recurred three years later, Louise had died in August 1985.

Although Rex and I had been living in Virginia at the time of her death, we had come to Provo and were able to visit with Louise and Larry shortly before she died. Louise's body had been ravaged by the cancer, but the beauty of her spirit shone through as we were with her for the last time, and I was struck by the artificiality of our worldly values as I saw eternity beckoning my friend. When I first walked into Louise's bedroom, I drew back in momentary horror before I was able to sit by her and talk. But as our visit continued, I was able to see and feel things beyond my mortal perceptions.

When we left the Wimmers' home after visiting that day, I was overcome with the impression that our being in Provo at this time was not by chance and that there were lessons I needed to learn from this visit with our friend. Now, two years later, Larry shared this thought with us: "Commonly, it is believed that there are winners and losers in the battle against cancer. Louise eventually died of her disease, but she did not lose. In life and in death, Louise was a winner who taught us how to live, how to suffer if that be our lot, and eventually how to die."

Reading Larry's words as my own husband struggled against cancer, I became all the more determined to fight our fight with the dignity and grace that I had seen in my friend Louise and that her husband later characterized with such eloquence.

Rex: Although I was unable to attend church during my first few months at NIH, I did benefit in very direct and meaningful ways from my ongoing associations with the Church. A very simple act that served as a great strength to me was partaking of the sacrament. Every Sunday afternoon, either the elders quorum from the nearby Bethesda ward or my former colleagues in the McLean ward high priests group would come to my room, close the door, and administer the sacrament to me.

I also had regular contact with my counselors in the Provo Oak Hills Third Ward, who called each Sunday morning to discuss ward business with me. I have no doubt that I was more of a bother to them than a help, although I was actively involved in calling a new Relief Society president and in reviewing all the other callings that needed to be decided. So whether I was of any real help or not, I found it very therapeutic to feel that I could still serve in the Church.

On one occasion, the ward recorded a sacrament meeting and sent the tape to Janet and me. One Sunday morning, Janet played the tape as I lay in bed, and before the opening song was finished, we were both wiping away tears. (In fact, to this day, I cannot hear that song without becoming quite emotional.) As we listened to the tape, I could envision myself sitting on the stand and looking out over the congregation, and that mental image became a great source of strength to me. The ongoing reminders that I was still the bishop gave me the hope that one day I could actually return to our ward and serve actively in that position.

The one significant involvement I had with the ward stemmed from a commitment I had made months earlier to speak in sacrament meeting. September 17, 1987, marked the two-hundredth anniversary of the ratification of the United States Constitution by the Constitutional Convention, and as a bishopric we had planned the previous spring to honor that occasion in a sacrament meeting. My counselors, George Bowie and Dave Jacobson, convinced me the ward was still expecting to hear from me, and we agreed that I would record a talk that could then be played in sacrament meeting.

Over several days, I recorded my talk on my little pocket recorder. But somehow I forgot I was dictating a talk rather than a letter, so I included each comma and period, as was my practice when dictating something that would then be transcribed. When George received the tape and heard what I had done, he didn't have the heart to send it back for me to redo. So somehow he had the tape doctored and removed each of the instances when I had said, "comma," "question mark," "semi-colon," and "period."

Toward the end of my stay at NIH, I asked for permission to leave the hospital and accompany Janet to church one Sunday. My oncologist, Dr. Rosenberg, was not a religious person himself, but he was convinced that people's religious beliefs (or something similar in the case of those who entertain no such beliefs) are essential in the healing process. He could understand, therefore, my wanting to go, but he set the condition that I have a blood test first and then call from the chapel two hours later to see if I needed to return to the hospital for a platelet transfusion. I made the call and learned that my platelet count had more than tripled. The next Sunday, when I was given permission to leave for a while and asked for instructions, Dr. Rosenberg said, "I have only one: Go to church."

Janet: As we moved toward autumn, Rex was responding well to the chemotherapy but still suffering from the infections that inevitably followed. I had felt that Christie might be better off staying in Washington, D.C., with me. Yet as September approached, I wasn't at all sure where I could send her to school (since we were not official residents of the area) and how I would juggle both her needs and Rex's.

Almost from the first day we were at NIH, Rex and I had received cards and letters from a former neighbor in Virginia, Nikii Frank. She was a lovely Christian woman who had a son close to Christie's age and a three-year-old daughter. When she learned Christie was living with me, she offered to have us move in with her. I, of course, did not want to impose, but as we got closer to the beginning of the school year, Nikii's offer seemed more and more to be a blessing I could not refuse.

We agreed that Christie and I would move in with the Franks on Saturday, August 29. As it turned out, Rex was very sick that morning, but I really had no choice except to leave him by early afternoon, return to our apartment to pack, load up Christie and all our belongings, and make the trip from Maryland to Virginia.

Even on a Saturday afternoon, the traffic on the Washington Beltway can be quite heavy, and this day was typical, with bumper-to-bumper cars traveling at about sixty-five miles an hour. Suddenly, about three car lengths ahead of me, I saw a stalled semitrailer in my lane. What immediately flashed into my mind was a report I had heard of a driver who had been decapitated by crashing into a stopped truck. I could tell I didn't have time to stop, so I swerved first to one side and then the other, at which point the car behind me hit me. That threw me back into the right lane and in the path of another car, which also hit me and sent my car into the median between two three-lane highways going in opposite directions. By the time I came to a stop, there were at least six other cars involved in the accident. My car was crushed to such an extent that Christie and I had to be pried out. Fortunately, neither of us was seriously hurt, but we were badly shaken by what had happened.

As the police were filling out their reports, I wondered how Christie and I were going to get ourselves—and all our belongings—to Nikii's house. I asked an officer if he could give me a ride to the nearest bus stop or telephone booth. He said no, they weren't allowed to do that. So I asked if I could at least use his phone, and he said no, they weren't allowed to do that either. He then explained that there were telephones every mile or so along the highway and that I could walk to one of those to make a call.

As my car was being hooked up to the tow truck and I was scrambling to get a few things out, the tow truck driver, seeing my plight, told me that while he couldn't take me wherever I needed to go, he could take me to where he was going and that there would be a phone there. So Christie and I rode with him to a telephone booth just outside the wrecking yard, where he helped us unload all our things onto the sidewalk.

When I called Nikii, she wasn't home (which seemed right

in line with how this day was going), but I was able to reach her at her mother's house, where Nikii's children were swimming. She told me she'd need a few minutes to change and about forty-five minutes to get to where we were, so Christie and I sat down on the curb just as it began to get dark. Nikii finally arrived, and as we loaded all of our belongings into her station wagon, I felt that she was the second angel of mercy to have helped us that day.

I didn't sleep well that night, but I got up early the next day because I wanted to see Rex before going to church. I put on my pink silk dress and high heels. Nikii loaned me her car, and I headed off for Maryland. About five miles out on the highway, I noticed yellow smoke billowing out of the car's hood, and then the car just died. Fortunately, the traffic was fairly light, and I was able to pull over to the side of the road without getting hit. From my experience the day before, I knew there was a phone no more than a mile away, so I took off down the highway to find it.

Before I had gotten very far, a man in his thirties, with two little children in the backseat, stopped and asked if I needed some help. He said, "I don't usually do this, but you don't look like someone who ought to be walking along the highway." And although I am generally not inclined to accept rides from strangers, at this point I was ready to make an exception to that rule. He took me to a gas station, where I arranged to have the car towed and repaired—and where I called one of those many friends who, through the entire four months Rex was in the hospital, had repeatedly come to our aid when we really needed it.

Within a few days, Christie and I had settled comfortably into the Frank home, where Nikii joined together with our longtime friends and former neighbors Margie and Jim Johnson in taking Christie into their families during the long hours that I was with Rex. Fortunately, I will never have to wonder how I would have managed without my friends' help.

Rex: The attitude I developed toward the hospital was an interesting mixture of feelings. By any standard, those four months
were far from pleasant. My world consisted largely of one small
room. On my periodic trips to nearby treatment rooms, I was
always accompanied by my IV pole. The food initially tasted just
like all other hospital food, but with the onset of my nausea I
learned to dread even the sound of the food cart coming down
the hall three times a day. The mere thought of food was posi-
tively repulsive to me.

Yet for all of the unattractive aspects of hospital life, I began
to develop not only an attraction for the place, but almost a
compulsive fear of being away from it. (I understand that this is
not an uncommon reaction for people who spend extended periods in hospitals or in other institutions, including prisons.) After
I had been at NIH for about two months, I was given permission
to leave for a few hours one evening. Janet and I brought some
Chinese food to her apartment and invited six of our good
friends to have dinner with us and visit. This was my first time
out, and there certainly were aspects of the experience that I
enjoyed (except for the food, which I couldn't handle any better
in Janet's apartment than I did in the hospital even though the
quality was considerably better). But all the time I was there, and
on subsequent occasions when I was given a pass to leave, I felt
somewhat insecure and was actually relieved when I could
return to my bed and my IV pole.

The one notable exception to this general feeling was when
I left the hospital on October 6 to argue a case before the United
States Supreme Court. Throughout my stay at NIH, Dr.
Rosenberg and others were very pleased with the fact that I was
working. In fact, the doctor soon began to include as one of his
standard questions during our daily visits, "Were you able to do
any work today?" My effectiveness varied from day to day, but I
was still productive enough that I was asked, during my stay, to
present the oral argument in a case involving the constitutional-
ity of "moments of silence" or "silent prayer" in public school
classrooms. Based on precedent, I was convinced that if we

could persuade the Court to reach the merits of the case, we would win. But there was a serious question whether the Court would reach the merits, because the member of the New Jersey legislature who had taken the case to the Supreme Court no longer held his position in the legislature and therefore arguably lacked "standing" to be a party to the case. Even with that potential problem with the case, I was ecstatic when the New Jersey lawyer who had taken the case to the Supreme Court asked me to argue it.

When the issue of my leaving the hospital for something as strenuous as a Supreme Court argument came up, my doctors were not quite as thrilled as they were about my working a few hours a day. I presented my case to them with vigor, however, explaining that the oral argument would last only half an hour and that this would be a real lift to me emotionally. They finally agreed, on the condition that I arrange with the Court to allow a nurse to accompany me (complete with a bagful of hypodermic needles and drugs to be administered, if necessary) and that the Court provide me with a stool that I could sit on if I became weak during the argument. These requests were an unusual accommodation for the Court, whose officers normally do not like to depart from standard procedures. But they graciously agreed and also offered me the use of my former haunt, the solicitor general's office at the Court, where I could rest for a few minutes before the Court session began. The clerk also scheduled me for the first argument in the morning, so that I wouldn't have to wait at the backup counsel table during earlier arguments.

The only remaining issue for me was whether I should appear in Court in my bald-as-a-billiard-ball state, the result of the chemotherapy, or wear one of my two hairpieces, which the full-service staff at NIH provided for each of its cancer patients. After the argument was scheduled and I had been given permission by NIH to go, my longtime friend Justice Anthony Scalia visited me at NIH. We enjoyed a nice social visit, and then I explained to him that while I knew we could not discuss anything relating to the merits of this case, I wondered if he would give me his opinion on whether I should wear my hairpiece or appear before the court completely bald. He responded that he thought I ought to wear the toupee because the other justices had not seen me with my very bald head and it might detract from what I had to say.

So the day of the argument, I choked down as much oatmeal as I could tolerate, was unhooked from my IV pole (although the needles remained in my arms), got dressed with Janet's help (complete with my toupee, which in hindsight I wish I hadn't worn), and was driven to the Court. My parents and my brother Mark were there, as well as Janet, several members of my firm, and other friends. The nurse from NIH sat directly behind me. The Court had indeed provided a stool for me to sit on, but after less than thirty seconds, my adrenaline was flowing and I knew I wouldn't need to sit down. And even though the Court ultimately ruled against us (which had more to do with the standing of our client than with my appearance), this experience, together with several others, helped me feel that I was still a contributing part of society. This feeling of worth gave me the ongoing and much-needed motivation to live.

Within days of my Supreme Court argument, I received another tremendous lift to my spirits when Dr. Rosenberg informed me one morning that after just three of the six chemotherapy cycles, my cancer was "in complete and unequivocal remission." Though the news was unexpected, those were wonderful words to hear. My doctor was quick to point out that remission does not mean cure, and the complete report he gave me included both good news and bad.

Because NIH is a research organization, all important decisions with respect to each patient are made by a group of doctors. The group assigned to my case had decided, Dr. Rosenberg explained, not to administer any more chemotherapy, both because I was in remission and because of the significant risk that my immune system could not withstand another cycle. So on the one hand, I was greatly relieved not to have to go through the nausea and other extreme illness that always accompanied the administration of these drugs. But I could tell, although he didn't say so directly, that Dr. Rosenberg had dissented from this decision; I believe he was fearful that while the drugs I had been given were sufficient to cause a remission, they were not sufficient to bring about a cure.

Even with this news, the doctors kept me at NIH throughout the remainder of October as an outpatient. I continued to receive radiation treatments, which were intended to diminish the chances of my cancer's return, and I completed my daily amphotericin-B treatments (the "ampho-terrible" drug used to rid my body of fungal infections).

Janet: I arrived at the hospital that morning just after Dr. Rosenberg gave Rex the news, and as I entered Rex's room I sensed that something good had happened. Rex was trying to restrain a tentative smile, and as I noticed a trace of tears in his eyes, he said to Dr. Rosenberg, "You tell her." But Dr. Rosenberg said, "No, I think you should be the one to tell her."

"Tell me what!" I asked, searching their eyes for an answer. Finally, too choked up to speak clearly, Rex managed to say, "I'm in remission."

I couldn't speak as I looked at his worn-out body and his bald head. Once strong, his body now had no muscle tone. His skin, once tanned and healthy, was now a pasty, grayish white. His face was swollen from prednisone, and his eyes had lost their shine. He was too weak to walk alone, and he still had IV fluids draining into both arms. The doctors had told us at the outset that the treatments would be almost unbearable. Rex's appearance reminded me of the truth of that statement.

"Isn't this wonderful?" he said as he waited for my reaction. When he spoke, I was jerked back to the moment.

"It *is* wonderful," I said. Then I managed a smile and kissed him, but I was well aware of my very tentative reaction and began to ask myself a long list of questions: Will there be more chemotherapy? How long will the remission last? Do I dare hope that the worst is over? If I get excited about our lives returning to normal, will I be hurt again?

I had never imagined that this would be my reaction. I had never understood pessimists who are afraid to hope the best, fearing that the worst will happen and they will then be disappointed. But I had been hurt so badly, and now I was at least surviving from day to day. I didn't want to let my spirits soar and then be hurt again. I knew that I had to be excited for him, for us, and for our family, but I needed first to rid myself of these fears.

It took several weeks before the reality of Rex's remission began to settle in. I found that as I told people the news, their happiness for us would lift my spirits as well, and I also learned that mine was not an unusual reaction, given our circumstances.

Perhaps more than anything, however, I overcame my hesitations as I expressed to Heavenly Father my gratitude for Rex and for the gift of his life. As I drove to the hospital one morning near the end of October, I spoke aloud in prayer, recounting the many blessings we had been given. As I did so, I realized that our happiness should not be restrained by the possibility of being hurt again. I had been grateful for each day before Rex's remission, and now with new hope, we faced a brighter future. I had cried many times while driving along the parkway, but this morning my tears flowed from my joy—and reflected a depth of gratitude I had never before known.

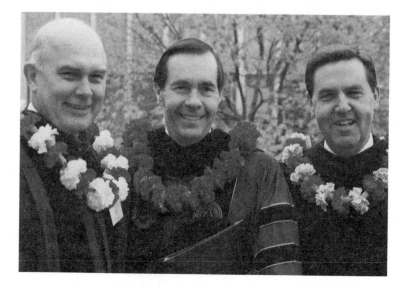

President Rex E. Lee is joined for his inauguration
by former BYU presidents Dallin H. Oaks (left)
and Jeffrey R. Holland.

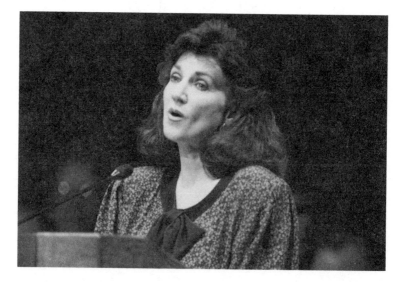

Janet addresses students in the first of many BYU devotionals,
September 1989.

CHAPTER 6

"All Is Well"

Janet: During the months that I sat by Rex's bedside, I watched
as he changed into someone who barely resembled my husband of almost thirty years. Physically, he was very weak and
emaciated and had no hair. But more significantly, he had lost
his independence as he came to rely on the NIH staff and me
to meet virtually all of his needs. One night in particular
demonstrated to me the extent to which our roles had been
redefined. My reflections on the incident caused me great concern as we prepared for him to leave the hospital.

Before I left the hospital each night, Rex and I would close
the door, say a prayer together, and then give each other a hug
and a kiss. One night, I had made my way through the ten-
minute maze of halls and elevators and was waiting on the
main floor for the parking elevator when a nurse found me

and said, "Your husband is calling for you." I hurried back to his room and asked what I could do to help him.

He responded, "You forgot to help me brush my teeth." Suddenly I saw with great clarity the completeness in the transformation of my once strong and self-sufficient husband into this frail and totally dependent cancer patient.

The idea of leaving the hospital, then, seemed like something of a mixed blessing. I was overwhelmed with gratitude that the doctors had deemed him well enough to leave, but I knew that without his intravenous feedings and the support of the NIH staff, he would have to rely on me for much of his care. The responsibility would be mine if anything went wrong. I was thrilled at the prospect of rebuilding our lives together, but we had just been through a rather radical transformation of our roles, with me taking over the job of managing all aspects of our lives—responsibilities which we had rather comfortably divided between the two of us during our marriage. I had never wanted to take this much control of our family matters, but I knew it would be months, maybe even years, before Rex would be completely better, able to take his former responsibilities again. This meant one more adjustment was ahead as we each defined and then assumed yet another new set of roles in our marriage.

In preparation for his leaving the hospital, I had rented a two-bedroom apartment in which Christie, Rex, and I stayed until we returned to Provo. Our first night there was complicated by the fact that Melissa had come for a brief visit and Michael, who was in Washington working as a senate page but living in the dorms provided for the pages, decided to bring two of his friends and spend the night.

The commotion combined with my concerns to make for a fitful night as I contemplated this change in our lives. For some reason, I had thought that the many lonely nights I had spent without Rex would be erased by his return, but the reason for his long absence came with us, and I feared it would come between us as well. Even lying next to him felt unfamiliar, and I spent many hours wondering what would be involved in rebuilding our lives and wishing he would awaken and tell me how he was feeling.

As I sought for spiritual strength and guidance, my thoughts turned to the deeper understanding I had gained of our Heavenly Father and his love for us. I certainly would not have chosen the events of the past four months as a way to learn the lessons I was learning, but at the same time I knew I was grateful for this part of our life together. Rex's cancer had presented us with a crash course in so many things, but the alternative to learning the lessons was failing the most important test I had ever been given. So while I wasn't quite sure how we would deal with what was ahead, I knew that with the Lord's help, we would find a way.

Rex: A recurring and overwhelming thought I had while in the hospital was how good life can be when we're well enough to enjoy it—and how desperately I wanted that opportunity once again. When I was too weak to stand up, I would wish for the chance to head out on a ten-mile run. When I was too sick to swallow, I would crave a hearty meal of soft-shell crabs or bean burritos. As each Sunday came, I would long to be with my fellow ward members back home in Provo. In short, my mind would often turn to life's basic pleasures, and I prayed for the day when I could partake of them once again.

So when the doctor told me on Wednesday, October 21, that I would be able to leave NIH the following Monday, I was thrilled—notwithstanding the fact that I would have to return each morning for radiation therapy, smaller doses of "amphoterrible," and platelet transfusions. It didn't take long, however, for me to realize how emotionally tied to the hospital I was, and on Sunday I spent considerable time contemplating my attachments to this place that had become my home. Nonetheless, I concluded, giving up my sense of security would more than be offset by living with Janet (even if we couldn't return to Provo just yet) and having the freedom to determine my own comings and goings.

I was also aware, as I thought about leaving, that while my cancer was in remission, there was the significant risk of a relapse. That was not something I liked to dwell on, although I knew I had to face that possibility. As I reviewed my condition—including all the statistical indications of my improved health (some of which were more encouraging than others)—the thing that gave me the greatest solace was reflecting on the words of President Bateman's blessing, which he did not qualify with percentages.

My first real outing after leaving NIH was to go trick-or-treating with Janet, Christie, several couples we knew, and their children. Throughout all our years together, this was something I had always done with our children, and I really wanted to go. We had brought so few of my clothes with us when we first came to NIH that Janet had to go buy me a shirt, jeans, jacket, gloves, and a hat to cover my still-bald head. It must have been obvious to many whose doors we knocked on that I was not well, as several gracious people asked if we would like to come in and sit down for a minute (this invitation is characteristic of Southern hospitality). Janet was slightly stunned the first time I said yes, but I simply did not have the stamina to make it around the neighborhood without sitting down occasionally.

After our night of trick-or-treating, my routine became one of spending my mornings in the hospital and my afternoons in my office at Sidley & Austin. Because my reflexes were not what they once were, Janet drove me everywhere. She handled with her usual grace and support my needing to be part of the world again.

Just after I was released from NIH, I had the second opportunity during those four months to appear before the Supreme Court. For several months, my friend Bruce Hafen, who was then dean of the BYU law school, had been arranging to bring a group of the school's graduates—my former students—back to Washington to be admitted to practice in the Supreme Court.

There are three ways to be admitted into the bar of this, the nation's highest court. The first is simply to file the necessary papers and pay the required fee by mail. The second is to have a lawyer who is already a member of the bar recommend an individual attorney's admission in open court. The third is the less common practice of a larger group of lawyers being introduced to the court by a single attorney. When this is done, the lawyer introducing the group simply reads the names of those to be admitted, as well as the state bar associations of which they are already members, and then says, "I am satisfied that each of them possesses the necessary qualifications." It is an absolute rule of the Court that you do not editorialize in making this presentation—that you stick right to the script. But on this morning, as I read the names of my friends to the nine justices and considered the fact that I was going to be able to return to my faculty position and the full-time practice of law, I was overwhelmed with emotion. So I bent the rules just a bit as I added, "Mr. Chief Justice, *these are my students.* I am satisfied that each of them possesses the necessary qualifications." Chief Justice William Rehnquist looked right up at me and then smiled from ear to ear, knowing full well what this moment meant to me.

Janet: Returning to Provo just days before Thanksgiving was very symbolic for me. Five months earlier, as we had backed out of our driveway, I had looked at the deep green leaves of our crab apple trees against the backdrop of the summer mountains and wondered whether Rex would return home with me. Now, as only a few brown leaves hung lifeless on bare branches, we were returning home to celebrate a holiday that had once represented a time to store up against the winter months ahead, as the frozen earth awaited the promise of spring.

That night I listened to the rhythm of Rex's breathing as we slept in our own bedroom for the first time in months, and I remembered my need to be grateful for newly appreciated blessings: enjoying the familiarity of our home and pleasant surroundings which brought unbelievable comfort; being able to cook in my own kitchen, with our family around me, and then washing familiar dishes; kneeling in family prayer; sitting on a child's bed and talking late into the night; writing at my desk or playing the piano. I wondered whether I had known such gratitude for these simple things the last time I had slept in this bed.

I smiled as I closed my eyes and thought again about the barren trees outside, and I considered that the symbol of my life was not to be found in these lifeless branches of the season, nor in the birds that had flown south to find sustenance in a less harsh climate. Instead, I knew that I could find my sustenance at home as I waited for the world to bloom again.

Just before Christmas, our ward had a surprise party for Rex, at which he was presented with a quilt that included the names of all the members of the ward. Each family had hand-embroidered a square of the quilt, which was then pieced together by skillful sisters and hand-quilted at various Relief Society and Young Women meetings. Sisters had gathered together in extra meetings in order to complete the project by our return home. The quilt was a huge undertaking, but we were told it had brought unity into the ward as all the members had fasted, prayed, and quilted.

Then on Christmas Day, we enjoyed what our children still regard as their very favorite Christmas, even though we didn't spend much on them or do anything particularly special. They were overjoyed just to have Rex home with the family again.

For me, however, the day involved mixed emotions. My sister, who by this time was divorced and had moved to Provo, spent part of the day with us, and late in the afternoon she began to play some of the songs on the piano that we had sung together over the years, both as children and adults. Almost immediately, I asked her to stop. I knew I had just been given the gift I most wanted, yet there was much about our situation that was very tentative, and my heart was still heavy. That was the one Christmas in my lifetime that I just could not sing.

In significant ways, being home was harder for me than being at NIH. There, Rex had an oncologist who watched over him constantly and a team of specialists who met each Friday to confer on his case. Now his care was my responsibility, and it frightened me that he was still so very weak. Rex is not always the best at monitoring his condition, and I knew that if I didn't watch him, no one would. That created in my mind the added burden that it would be my fault if something happened to him, and I worried about him constantly. Then, late one night in early January, the moment arrived that I had feared. Rex began to run a high fever, which signaled some kind of infection.

The only thing I could think to do was call NIH. I was told to get Rex to our local hospital and have the doctors in Provo administer an antibiotic intravenously. Rex was in the hospital for four days while the doctors got his infection under control, and during that time we were very worried, both of us being well aware that one of the principal causes of death among cancer patients—either present or former—is pneumonia.

Rex: As concerned as I was about taking care of myself, I felt a real need to be productive, at least for a few hours a day. Doing so required quite an adjustment, as I moved back into a life where I wasn't tied to a hospital room. My inclination, of course, was to start spending most of my time at my office. Janet, on the other hand, thought I should have a period of transition during which I spent the majority of my time at home resting. The net result was a compromise, though at the time I thought the compromise was mostly toward her view, while she thought just the opposite.

Even with focusing on my work, however, the single factor that dominated my thoughts—and Janet's as well—was the possibility that my cancer would return. I did take comfort in the fact that before long I could work six or seven hours a day and that my blood counts were returning to a respectable level. But I continued to dread my monthly checkups at NIH—partly because of the memories that returned as I got off the subway and walked toward the facility and partly because I was afraid of what the doctors might find. Each time that I went, the news was good, and I would leave the building with a sense of enormous relief as I headed back toward the subway.

My emotional reactions to that building were so irrational that I continued to be amazed by my feelings, even though I was told they were completely typical. I literally developed a love-hate relationship with the place. On the one hand, I was grateful to the people and the facilities for the role they had played in preserving my life. But as I drew closer to the building from the subway on the occasion of each of my monthly visits, my anxieties increased, and it was all I could do to force myself to open the door and go in. Then when I left, I would almost literally run.

In late March 1988, I made my first trip back to NIH without Janet. I didn't think I could be any more aware of how much she had done for me over the previous nine months, but on that trip, I saw her in a whole new light. Quite literally, I felt like half a person while I was away from her, and I realized how much I had depended on her and how much strength I had derived from having her with me. As much as I missed her, it was perhaps good for me to have this realization renewed.

During my day alone at NIH, I also reflected at length on the contrast between my life as an inpatient and all that I could enjoy with my cancer in remission. My sense of appreciation for the finite segments of life had greatly increased since the previous June. Days, weeks, and months had once melted together in my mind, but now each moment had great meaning to me. And while I would never recommend cancer as a way of increasing one's level of appreciation for life's simple moments, it certainly did have that effect on me.

Within days of this trip, our home teachers came for one of their regular visits. Their lesson involved the importance of keeping the companionship of the Holy Ghost at all times and not doing anything that would impede the Spirit's influence. Their message brought to my mind that one of life's great ironies—even tragedies—is that it is harder to maintain the Spirit when times are good than when times are difficult. That Sunday afternoon, I reflected on the fact that while the chances of my cancer returning were still high, so many things had returned to "normal" that it was increasingly easier for me to let things spiritual fall into the background of my life.

Beginning in June, I couldn't help but think each day about what had happened on each particular day the year before: becoming aware of my fatigue, "injuring" my back, receiving my doctor's initial diagnosis, traveling to NIH for treatment, and enduring the four months of chemotherapy. The contrast of those memories with the present was marked. Even though I still was not feeling completely better, I could go to work each day, I could spend time with my family, and I could serve as bishop—although my counselors continued to carry more than their fair share of the load. And after having exercised by walking for several months, I could even run a little bit most days.

June 25 was especially memorable. That was the one-year anniversary of the day on which the doctors in Provo had definitely confirmed the cancer (after our return from Boise) and on which I began telling my children, parents, and friends of my condition. On this day in 1988, I remembered back to a time at NIH when Janet had told me one of her fondest hopes. "I will be so glad," she said to me, "when the day comes that I can ask you how you're feeling and your response will be, 'I feel great.'"

That afternoon, as I returned home from the law school, I reminded Janet of her comment from the previous year (which she remembered well). Then I said, "I'm not quite there yet, but I'm getting *very* close!"

By early August, the most obvious reminder of my cancer was the fact that I couldn't run any faster than a ten-minute mile, although my pre-cancer rate had been an eight-minute mile or better. The other reminder, to which I had grown accustomed, was a constant ringing in my ear, which I had experienced ever since I left the hospital. These were minor considerations, given that I was enjoying a full life once again—and had even been able to hold up during a three-day river trip with the youth in our ward. A week later, when we held a family reunion with my side of the family, I couldn't help but remember that the year before at this time, I wasn't at all sure I would outlive my parents.

Perhaps the culminating moment of these reflections on the previous year came while we were in Washington, D.C., for my quarterly checkup at NIH and for an argument before the United States Court of Appeals for the District of Columbia. Janet and I spent our last night there with our friends Dee and Patti Benson, Jim and Margie Johnson, and Jim and Bette Jo Croft. We ate Chinese food and watched a BYU football game, as the eight of us had done almost one year to the day earlier. There were two big differences this time, however. First, whereas a year earlier BYU had been massacred by Pitt, this year they beat the University of Texas, 47–6. And second, whereas in 1987 I had spent most of the night in the bathroom throwing up, this time I was able to enjoy the meal.

All in all, things were going very well, which is to say that I felt good about everything.

Janet: As the months moved on, Rex became stronger and stronger, and the day finally did come when he could say, without equivocation, "I feel great." Sometimes as we were together I would study my handsome husband. He looked young again. His hair was as thick as ever, without a gray strand in it. His skin had regained its youthful glow, and his step had its old, familiar bounce. His eyes were clear and sparkling, and his voice was strong. There simply were no traces of the body that had once been wracked by cancer and chemotherapy.

He was running again, as well as teaching at the law school and enjoying his long-distance partnership with Sidley & Austin. We were getting our feet back on the ground financially and our family back together emotionally. As the early months of 1989 moved along, life was finally beginning to seem a little less tentative.

On Friday, April 7, Rex and I were in Arizona to attend a BYU Law Society dinner. We were staying in Mesa with my parents, and that evening, as we were rushing to get ready (actually, Rex was rushing me), the telephone rang. When my dad told Rex the phone was for him, Rex said, "You go get in the car, and I'll be right there." It was a familiar request to save time, but in Mesa's heat, I wasn't anxious to oblige him. As I waited in the house, Rex went into the study and then shut the door. Although we were running late, he stayed in there for several minutes.

When he came out, I said, "Who was that? I thought we were in a hurry?" He answered in a hushed tone as we walked out of the door with my parents: "It was Elliot Cameron, and I'll talk to you about it later." As we drove to the dinner, Rex and I made small talk, but all the way there I kept thinking, "Elliot Cameron. Elliot Cameron. I know that name." I knew he had a Church connection, but I could not quite put him in the right context.

We sat at the dinner with my parents, as well as our daughter Diana and her husband, Steve. Halfway through the salad course, an alarm went off inside my head as I remembered that Elliot Cameron was the commissioner of Church education. I began wondering why he would be calling Rex— and why the call had made him so nervous—and suddenly it dawned on me. Jeffrey R. Holland, who had been president of BYU since 1980, had been called the previous Saturday to the Church's First Quorum of the Seventy, which meant the position of BYU president needed to be filled. Rex's reaction to the telephone call made me wonder if he was being considered for the position.

Later that night, when we were alone, Rex explained to me that the call was to elicit his help in finding a new president. That explanation helped me relax somewhat although not completely. Rex never applied or asked to be considered for positions. Things just dropped in his lap unexpectedly, and my concern as we talked was that this might be one of those moments. The only thought I had ever given to that position was when Rex would comment, based on his associations with Presidents Oaks and Holland, that being president of BYU was "a killer of a job." The idea that it might one day fall to Rex had never been an issue in my mind.

Rex: The specific purpose of Commissioner Cameron's call was to ask me to meet the following Tuesday at 8:30 A.M. with the search committee that had been appointed to recommend a successor to Elder Holland. That committee was composed of Elders Marvin J. Ashton (who chaired the committee), L. Tom Perry, and Neal A. Maxwell. Frankly, I thought of little else other than my upcoming appointment between Friday night and Tuesday morning.

Although Commissioner Cameron had not stated this explicitly, I knew enough of the workings of such committees to conclude that I was likely being considered as one of several candidates for the position. As I considered this possibility, I felt some ambivalence. On the one side of the ledger, I felt nothing but great love and loyalty for BYU, and this position would be the ultimate relationship of service to this wonderful university. On the other side, I was very much enjoying what I was presently doing. I was pretty good at practicing law, and I didn't know whether I would be a good university president or not. Furthermore, as I had expressed to Janet on various occasions, being BYU president would be, indeed, a killer of a job—not only because of the sheer volume of the workload but also because of the many publics with whom the president must deal, with no single one of them having expectations identical to those of the others.

Before my meeting with the search committee, Janet and I discussed our views openly and thoroughly. Her reaction was pretty much the same as mine, although she expressed it better: We would approach this with some trepidation and almost hope that it would not be offered to us. But if it was offered, there would be no way we could say no, particularly in view of my newfound health. My additional view on the matter was that I had absolutely no control over how this would all unfold, so I figured I might as well just sit back and see what happened on Tuesday morning.

My interview with the search committee, which lasted about forty minutes, was interesting. We talked about BYU, including its current status, what its future should be, and what steps should be taken to secure that future. But the principal focus of the interview was my health. I told them that if they put that question to my physicians, they would get an answer that was guarded and mixed. My cancer was in remission but could certainly return, especially since my chemotherapy treatments had been cut short. But though the doctors were uncertain about whether I would be present on this planet for the next several years, I was not, and I told them about the blessing I had received from President Bateman—and what a great, reassuring solace that blessing had been for me.

Interestingly, on the Friday following my interview, a rumor ran rampant across the BYU campus that I was going to be named the new president that afternoon. When people asked me about this story, I told them truthfully that I knew nothing about it—and that if such an announcement were made, I would be the most surprised person in attendance.

Janet: Near the end of March, we went to Mexico on a much-needed four-day vacation with Steve and Dixie Oveson, LaVell and Patti Edwards, and Ray and Debbie Goodson. We rested, swam in the ocean, ran, slept, and ate; but the warm, cordial conversations were the best part of the trip. Somewhere in our many talks, the question came up about who might be the next president of BYU. Someone suggested that Rex must have some inside information, but he simply said he didn't know, named a few possibilities, and then turned the conversation to another topic.

During our time there, I began to think more seriously about the possibility that Rex might be appointed, but my hope was that we could continue on in our present mode. I just wanted life to get back to normal—whatever that was—and not have to take on any additional responsibilities. Teaching school with a big family had been hard, moving back to Provo had been hard, and living through Rex's battle with cancer had been the hardest. What I wanted more than anything right then was a life that was a little easier.

One afternoon during our stay, I began to feel guilty about my selfish desires, and I reflected on my supplications to the Lord during Rex's illness. I had told my Heavenly Father repeatedly that I would go anywhere and do anything with Rex if he was allowed to remain with me. At the time, I had envisioned going on a mission and living in a little thatched hut in Africa, with bugs crawling all over us. In my estimation, having Rex with me would have more than made up for the discomfort.

Remembering my earlier resolve, I went into our bedroom overlooking the ocean and knelt in prayer. I told the Lord that I didn't want to stand in the way of whatever he wanted Rex to do and that if BYU was to be my African hut, then so be it. I committed anew that I would willingly do anything asked of me, with love and appreciation for Rex's precious gift of life. I arose from that prayer, moved beyond what I would have anticipated. In fact, I cried a little at the giving of my will to a greater power than mine. Or perhaps what moved me was not so much relinquishing my control as it was recognizing the power of the Lord. But I felt better, knowing that I would not resist whatever Rex was asked to do.

My complete submissiveness to the Father's will led to a strong, peaceful feeling: not one of being led against my will, but a feeling of strength being conveyed through my willingness to do our Father's bidding. As I left the bedroom, I concluded that I would have to wait and see what the Lord wanted us to do. Then I set the experience aside and enjoyed the rest of the vacation.

We returned home on Monday, and just as our plane touched down on the runway in Salt Lake City, I knew what was ahead. It was as strong a feeling as I have ever had. I was exhilarated and frightened at the same time, and I didn't sleep much that night. Never during our time in Mexico or on our first night home did we discuss the possibility that Rex might be called as the university president, but I was not surprised when Rex called the next morning to tell me that the First Presidency wanted to meet with the two of us on Thursday at 8:00 A.M.

Rex: Our interview with the First Presidency was fascinating, reminiscent of the interview we had with President Harold B. Lee in 1971 when I was asked to be the first dean of the J. Reuben Clark Law School. On both occasions we were told that these BYU positions are not Church callings; rather, they are offers of professional employment. Yet in both instances, we were told that a committee of General Authorities had considered the matter carefully and prayerfully and had come to the conclusion that I was the person the Lord wanted to serve. Though I accepted their explanation that this offer was different than a calling, I also knew that this was not something that a loyal, believing Church member would decline. Nor would I have done so had the matter been put to me as a straightforward offer of employment. Janet and I had already crossed that threshold, and I accepted gratefully and enthusiastically, though not without some misgivings about my own abilities, which I explained to the Brethren.

During this period, I was especially grateful to Janet for the reassurance and support she gave to me. I knew that the rewards would be largely mine and the sacrifices largely hers. But she was wonderfully supportive as she told the First Presidency of her promise to the Lord to support me in anything he wanted me to do. As for me, I had much the same feeling after our interview that I had experienced when I was asked to be solicitor general—both a thrill and a sense of unreality that such a thing was happening to me, a kid from St. Johns. With the government appointment, I was humbled by the fact that I was following legal giants such as John W. Davis, Robert H. Jackson, and William Howard Taft. This time my predecessors were spiritual and educational giants: Karl G. Maeser, George H. Brimhall, Franklin S. Harris, to name but three, as well as the three presidents I had personally known and admired—Ernest L. Wilkinson, Dallin H. Oaks, and Jeffrey R. Holland.

We did not tell our children what was happening until the day the announcement was made, but they knew I was being considered and pestered us with questions just the same. We were as evasive as we could be without prevarication, but it was particularly hard one morning when Melissa said to Janet, "Mom, I'm really glad Dad made the last cut. I just hope he doesn't make the next one." At that point, it was hard not to break the news to her: Unless some change occurred, I had made the final cut.

Janet: As we left the First Presidency's office, we were stunned as we began to consider the implications of what was ahead for us. At the same time, this opportunity seemed so right to me when I considered the events of the previous two years. To me, it seemed obvious that this was the reason Rex's life had been preserved (even though he has never been willing to acknowledge that such was the case). And it also struck me with great force that this was a job the Lord wanted us to do. *Us.* It felt so good to approach a job together, and I wanted to be a part of everything he did. I had nursed Rex back to health, and now I wanted to reap the harvest with him.

For Rex, working is his life's blood. I knew, as he recovered from the cancer, that he would always work—and work hard. I accepted that, yet I knew his focus typified the fact that we did things so differently. He wanted to plan each minute of his day by the clock, while I was more inclined to adapt my schedule as situations arose; he gave little thought to minor details, while I worried about such things perhaps more than was necessary; he was inclined to do two things at once, while what I wanted was his undivided attention when we talked. The very traits we found frustrating in each other were the same traits that, when manifest in other ways, became the most endearing. I loved his efficiency and was constantly amazed at how much he could accomplish. My painstaking attention to detail often pleased him when he saw the end result. We found that it worked best for us to smile through our differences and simply accept the total package. Looking toward BYU, I sensed that this new opportunity would enable us to enjoy in new ways the fact that our differences overlapped to make us who we were. And I could also see that this new opportunity would provide us with more time to be together than we had ever experienced before. I was profoundly grateful, once again, for how well the Lord knows each of us and how he blesses us individually.

As we prepared for Rex to assume his new responsibilities on July 1, 1989, I felt a surge of energy and almost giddy expectation brought on by being able to look beyond tomorrow. When we met with some of Rex's staff in a calendaring meeting just before he formally took office, I savored the chance to write specific commitments on my calendar—events that would take place a week, a month, six months ahead. It felt so good to see a life ahead of us, a life we would share after having lived so tentatively for the previous two years.

I wondered, as I left the meeting, how apparent my joy was to those on Rex's staff whom I was just getting to know. Then, as I drove out of the parking lot, I heard the Carillon Bells on campus mark a new hour with their familiar refrain from "Come, Come Ye Saints." As I listened, I remembered many times in the preceding months when I would hear those bells and my thoughts would turn to the line, "And should we die before our journey's through." But this afternoon I could only hear the glad refrain, "All is well! All is well!"

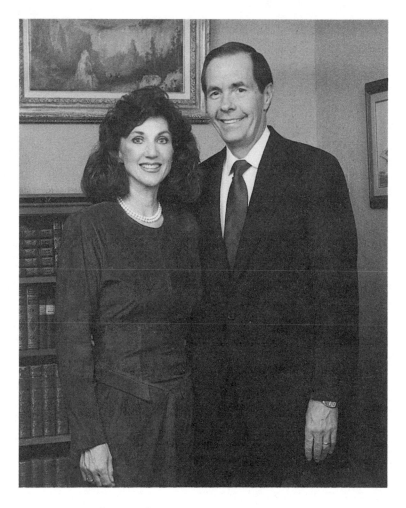

REX AND JANET POSED FOR THIS PORTRAIT
SOON AFTER REX'S APPOINTMENT AS PRESIDENT OF BYU IN 1989.

CHAPTER 7

Joy Defies Circumstances

Rex: From the very first day, I found my new job at BYU absorbing, interesting, and exciting. In part, my reaction stemmed from being so intimately involved with a university I have loved since I was eighteen years old. I also enjoyed finding new challenges and opportunities each day when I came to work. As my colleagues and I worked on issues and initiatives that we hoped would benefit the university, I enjoyed a resurgence in my energy level that I had not experienced since before my battle with cancer two years earlier. I was quick to recognize that, in large measure, the source of my newfound energy was a substance called adrenaline. I knew it wouldn't last forever, but for the moment, it sure beat chemotherapy.

More than anything else, though, the source of my enjoyment in this job was that Janet was so much a part of it. She literally shared in my responsibilities every day. There were the obvious events that brought us together—banquets, football and basketball games, concerts, receptions, and the like, which a president and his wife will typically attend together. But beyond that, Janet became very involved with the students, faculty, and alumni and shared with me the insights she gained from those interactions. I was filled with appreciation for all her qualities as we shared the social aspects of this new position as well as its challenges and burdens.

As the school year started in September 1989, Janet and I were feeling very optimistic about my health and my future prospects of health. We were on our first major trip for BYU, a trip that included fund-raising and other alumni activities in New York and Washington, D.C., and a football game between BYU and Navy (which we won). During the Washington segment of that trip, I made one of my quarterly visits to NIH, and the doctor said everything looked good. Janet then reminded him that it had been two years almost to the day since I had gone into remission, and we asked if that was a significant fact. His response was that for non-Hodgkins T-cell immunoblastic lymphoma, two years from the time of remission is *the* critical time and that only 10 percent of patients who reach that point go into relapse thereafter. I always experienced significant joy as I walked out of NIH's Building 10 following one of my checkups, but that day I almost floated out.

That prognosis was at the forefront of my consciousness for many days to come, and my thoughts centered on two things I had learned from my experience two years earlier. The first was the constant, everyday appreciation I felt for the privilege of participating in this earthly experience—which was a feeling that I knew would never diminish, no matter how many years passed after my bout with cancer. The second was my appreciation for Janet. Her loving care had benefited me throughout my life, but that was certainly highlighted during my months at NIH, as she had cared for me in ways that I would never forget. In fact, it is something of an understatement to say that no other human being could have been as good for me during that time as Janet was.

The months that followed that visit were filled with opportunities to view distinct parts of the university in ways I had never experienced them, to discuss with our board of trustees long-range issues facing the university, to meet with students and faculty in question-answer sessions, to participate in the inaugural ceremony held in my honor on October 27, to enjoy football and basketball games, and to visit with alumni and friends of the university. And if the fall hadn't been busy enough, as Janet and I looked ahead to the first few months of 1990, we saw a slate of activities that would keep us as busy as I had been since January through April of 1987. (Of course, I was not anxious to repeat the aftermath of those four months.)

Janet: Rex approached his new assignment at BYU with his characteristic passion and energy. In fact, his two secretaries, Janet Calder and Jan Nelson, commented to me almost immediately that they were astounded by the volume of work he could get through in a day and by the efficient way that he handled the various aspects of his job. They learned that they could almost set their clocks by his comings and goings, and others who worked with him soon discovered that they couldn't be late for a meeting or luncheon because he was always there on time. Having watched him work for the thirty years of our marriage, I was not surprised by people's observations on his performance. What did surprise me was the extent to which I was able to be part of his very busy life, which helped me enjoy every facet of our new life together. The university kept us busy, but we were also able to keep up with our always-active family, and we attended reunions, weddings, Fourth of July celebrations, grandchildren's birthdays, video parties, Sunday dinners, and Lake Powell vacations.

Just three weeks after Rex began his presidency, our granddaughter, Jordon, was born to Tom and Kimberly. Eighteen months later they increased our grandchildren to four with the addition of Jacob Rex. Also in 1991, Diana and Steve had their third child, Alexander Steven, and Wendy and Tom had their first, Colton Thomas. Grandparenting became a priority along with our other responsibilities.

My one fear, as the first few months rolled past, was the idea of speaking at the fall 1989 devotional in front of thousands of students as well as television cameras. But in the end I found the process of preparing that first talk to be quite invigorating. Then Rex suggested that at the January 1990 devotional we should talk about our experience with his cancer. That was not something I cared to do; I didn't want to expose so much personal pain. But Rex won out, and we worked together on the first of several talks that we would give side by side rather than one after the other.

A week before this devotional, we were at NIH for Rex's quarterly checkup. During that visit, the doctor expressed concern over an unusual spot on Rex's skin, as well as over some lymph nodes he could feel under Rex's left arm. It was agreed that Rex should submit to a biopsy of the spot when we returned to Provo. As we returned to Provo to put the finishing touches on our talk, we were feeling a great deal of apprehension about this rather uncertain situation. However, we didn't tell anyone about our experience at NIH, largely because we didn't know if there was any real cause for concern. As we concluded our talk, we explained that his cancer had, in fact, been the most important test we had ever been given—and he then added, "And it may not be finished yet." At that moment I experienced the ominous feeling of storm clouds gathering.

Rex: Near the end of January, Dr. Warren Eyre, who was then my dermatologist, did the biopsy on my skin just above the left elbow. He told me that it would be about a week before the results would be available. I explained that we would be in California for a few days and he suggested that I phone his office for the results.

As instructed, I made the phone call on Friday, February 9. Dr. Eyre was not in, but the nurse read me the analysis. To my great relief, the report was that I had psoriasis. That relief was shattered when I returned to Dr. Eyre's office the following Tuesday for a regularly scheduled appointment. He said that further analysis by a pathologist in Salt Lake had shown that the original diagnosis was wrong. Dr. Eyre then said, "This shows definite signs of T-cell involvement." Those precise words, like two other phrases before them—"definitely destructive lesions" and "complete and unequivocal remission"—will always remain with me. I immediately knew the significance of his words. They were tantamount to a death sentence. The treatments of most cancers are significantly more difficult the second time, and given my particular circumstances—including the type of cancer, this relapse after remission, and my compromised immune system—any attempted treatment would have to be characterized as a very long shot. Dr. Eyre informed me that his office had sent the analysis to Dr. J. Cordell Bott, my local oncologist, to compare these tests with those from my earlier diagnosis in 1987.

The next three days, Tuesday morning through Friday noon, were probably the darkest and most depressing of my life. I had asked Dr. Eyre to notify the people at NIH, and on Wednesday, I called my attending oncologist there and asked if he had heard the news. The response I received was phrased in the worst possible words, at least for me. He said, "Yes, I've heard. And I feel just terrible for you."

He of course meant well and was merely trying to express his sympathy. But sympathy has never been what I have wanted or needed. (That has been true since my cancer was first diagnosed in 1987.) What I really needed to hear that day was something like what I had been told almost three years earlier by Dr. Longo: "I want you to know that we're going to do everything we possibly can for you. I'm working on it right now, and I assure you we will leave nothing undone that can be done."

On Thursday afternoon, I was in a faculty advisory council

meeting in the law building when my friend and former assistant Carolyn Stewart came into the room and handed me a note to call Dr. Bott. I was terrified to make the call, and it was actually physically difficult for me to pick up the telephone and dial Dr. Bott's number. The news that he gave me was the worst possible, exactly what I had feared: "The markers on this most recent test match up closely with those from the tests we did in 1987." I asked him if he had reported those results to my oncologist at NIH. He said that he had, and they wanted to see me in Bethesda as soon as I could get there.

That was the lowest point of the entire three days. I imagined reentering the NIH hospital, probably never to emerge again until it became apparent to everyone—as it certainly would within a short time—that nothing else could be done for me, and I would then be sent home to die.

On Friday morning, we had a meeting in my office with Elders David B. Haight and James E. Faust on a university matter that had implications for the Church. At the conclusion of that meeting, I explained to these two brethren what had happened to me during the preceding three days, and I asked if they would be willing to administer to me. Elder Faust did the anointing, which was sealed by Elder Haight, with members of my president's council also participating in the circle. Elder Haight's blessing was quite different from the one I had received from Merrill Bateman three years earlier. His was basically a plea with the Lord to let me live. But it was not just an ordinary plea. It was stated and restated in several different ways, with an urgency in his voice that I had seldom heard.

After the blessing was over and these two brethren and my colleagues had left, my secretary, Janet Calder, told me that I'd had several phone calls and that the one from my friend Steve Freestone, director of pathology at Utah Valley Regional Medical Center, seemed particularly important. I returned Steve's call. His news was as welcome as it was unexpected. His partner, Paul Urie, who is an expert on a form of T-cell lymphoma called mycosis fungoides, had been reexamining the samples from my skin biopsy. He was virtually certain that what I had was not a relapse of my former immunoblastic lymphoma but rather this thing called mycosis fungoides. It is also a T-cell lymphoma, but in several respects it lies at the opposite end of the spectrum from the cancer I had in 1987. It was incurable, but indolent, and it could frequently be controlled. Steve told me that if I had this kind of cancer, they could predict a longer life expectancy than the very short time I could expect with a relapse of the immunoblastic form. He told me I could live for a fairly long time and, best of all, lead a pretty normal life.

I could scarcely believe my ears. I wanted to ask several questions, all at the same time. "Are you telling me," I asked, "that Janet and I can still take our planned trip to Jerusalem in a couple of months, that I can carry on my activities as president of BYU, and that I can run on Saturday mornings with Janet and my children?"

"Yes," he replied. "That's exactly what I'm telling you."

"How sure are you about Dr. Urie's diagnosis?" I asked.

He answered, "We're very certain. We've looked at it many times, and rather carefully, because while immunoblastic forms of T-cell lymphoma frequently follow the indolent forms, we don't know of any instance in which it has been in this order. But Paul is an expert on mycosis fungoides, and he is confident that that is what you have."

And then I asked the big question: "You say that I can expect to live for some time. What's your best guess as to how long that is?"

He responded that that would depend on a number of other factors, which had not yet been ascertained, but he would expect it to be years rather than months.

"How many years?" I asked.

Again, he responded, "That's impossible to answer with any degree of certainty and depends on a number of other as-yet-undetermined facts. But mycosis fungoides patients generally live between three and thirteen years following diagnosis."

I hung up the phone and sat there for some time, basking in

the joy of what my friend had told me. Perspective is an amazing thing. Four days earlier, if a doctor had informed me that I had an incurable form of cancer and could expect to live somewhere between three and thirteen years, I would have been devastated. But as I compared this news against the background of the earlier indications, I was ecstatic. My life was not about to come to an end, at least not within the next few months. If their diagnosis was correct, I could expect to see another Christmas. Indeed, many Christmases. I would be around for Michael's missionary farewell the following fall, and probably for his homecoming, and perhaps several weddings—not only Michael's but Stephanie's, Melissa's, and Christie's as well. And my life would be conducted outside of a hospital, doing normal things, including living with my family, continuing to work at a job that I enjoyed as much as any that I had ever had, and in general, leading a normal life. My greatest hope was that Dr. Urie's diagnosis would turn out to be correct.

When I called my oncologist at NIH, he told me that this diagnosis could not possibly be correct. He, of course, had had much more experience with T-cell lymphomas. And he said that the immunoblastic form always followed the indolent form, and it never happened the other way. For some reason, at that point I assumed the role of a fool—a lawyer who represents himself—and attempted to argue my case that I had mycosis fungoides. My approach was totally irrational, based on an assumption that if I could persuade this doctor, against his own judgment, I would somehow win an acquittal.

Janet: I was still in California, where I had stayed for a few extra days with our daughter, Wendy, after learning that Rex's biopsy showed nothing serious. When Rex returned to Provo and received the news we had both feared for two years, he decided to shield me from the turmoil he was undergoing until I returned home. But before Rex received Dr. Urie's report, his desperation overtook his desire to protect me, and he finally called to share with me what he had been told.

Courageously, he tried to explain the good in this bad news, and as I struggled to match his optimism, I did my best to give what comfort I could over the telephone—all the while thinking, *This cannot happen to us again.*

Neither of us nor our children had completely recovered from his first bout with cancer, and being hit with this second assault was unthinkable. As we talked, I thought of our children having to endure such grief again and wondered why Rex's job was now going to be made so difficult. As we poured out our hearts across the miles of telephone lines, we began to find relief, and finally I dried my tears as we began to plan for another battle with illness.

When we received the news that the biopsies showed an indolent form of cancer rather than the more aggressive form, which appeared to still be in remission, we had decided that the children needed to be told what was happening. We didn't want them to learn about Rex's cancer from some other source, and Rex needed to return to NIH immediately for tests.

Early Saturday morning, Rex began the task of talking with our children by waking Michael, who was then eighteen. Michael's initial reaction when Rex sat down on the side of the bed was that his father was going to make some sort of deal with him—probably that Michael clean the garage in the morning so that the two of them could do something together in the afternoon. When our son learned that his father had a second form of cancer, his first thought was that it was too much to hope for another miracle and that he would possibly lose his father before leaving on his mission—and most certainly before he returned.

Most of Michael's questions were answered with "I don't know," and in the absence of any concrete information, the two of them hugged, exchanged their love for each other, and shed more than a few tears.

That evening, Diana, Michael, Stephanie, Melissa, and Christie joined Rex for what he was determined would be a celebratory dinner. There the family discussed Rex's condition, and Rex assured them that this particular cancer would be slow to take his life. But because they had not gone through the sequence of events that Rex and I had, the children found it difficult to see this news as a cause for celebration. When Rex and the children returned home from dinner, they continued to talk about this turn of events, and then I called from California and talked with each child over the telephone. Many of their concerns were understandable: Why did we get Dad back only to have him taken again? Can we really expect another miracle? Will the two of you have to stay at NIH for a long time? Will Dad be here to write to me on my mission? Will he live long enough to know my children? How can I grow up without a father?

It took time for the fears to subside—partly because of the shock that inevitably accompanies such news and partly because Rex and I still had to return to NIH for more tests needed to confirm the nature of this second cancer. But finally we as a family found solace for our pain, and we chose to soothe our swollen eyes with thoughts of gratitude and hope.

Rex: Janet and I spent most of the next week at NIH, where people conducted the same tests and others as well. At the end of the week, the doctors rather incredulously came to the conclusion that Dr. Urie was right. They also told me that the country's leading expert on this particular form of cancer was Dr. Steven Rosen, a member of the medical faculty at Northwestern University, and that they would attempt to persuade him to take me on as a patient.

Dr. Rosen, in addition to being an expert on mycosis fungoides, is one of the finest human beings I have ever known. From the very first, we liked him as a doctor, as a person, and as a friend. He has the ability to recruit his patients' efforts in the process of their own healing.

In our first visit, he explained that while my disease is a lymphoma and not a skin cancer, it manifests itself in skin lesions, which can be one indicator of the progression of the cancer. In my case, however, the disease had reached my bone marrow, and Dr. Rosen decided I should skip the initial treatments and move to interferon injections, which are used when this cancer reaches a more advanced stage. Even though this could have been discouraging news, he gave it to us in such a positive context that I was not discouraged.

Janet: On February 26, 1990, our fifteen-year-old daughter, Melissa, made the following entry in her journal:

> *I found out something very disturbing tonight. My dad's cancer is incurable. There is no cure! They are working on one but as of now there isn't one. How could this be happening? He had cancer already two years ago. I thought we were through with this for years. This means my children won't know my dad, their grandpa. This is the saddest thought. I love my dad so much and want him to be around forever, not die in ten years, or less. He is announcing about his cancer to BYU tomorrow at 3:00. If you couldn't tell, I'm very upset right now and I'm going to go to bed.*

Rex concluded that he needed to tell the BYU community about his condition, and that announcement took place on February 27, his fifty-fifth birthday. The announcement itself was a difficult moment for me, but as I watched Rex share this news with the university family, I was struck once again by his love of life, by how deeply he can drink from the stream of life, and by how contagious his characteristic enthusiasm can be.

His style of leadership was evident as he encouraged the university to continue moving forward rather than being weighed down by this news, and I found myself lifted as well, knowing that he and I would have more time together—time I knew we would live in the fullest manner possible as we fought this new battle.

It was a battle we fought hard. Rex endured drugs and treatments, and at times we both experienced fear over what was ahead. But there were also very obvious blessings. One came in the form of outstanding medical care, provided by doctors who were determined to do all they could to keep this cancer in check. The interferon treatments Dr. Rosen prescribed lasted for almost two years. The shots were administered at home intermuscularly; half the time Rex would give them to himself in the abdomen, and the rest of the time, I would give them to him in the arm. From the very beginning, every indication was that the interferon did what it was supposed to. Indeed, during the time Rex took the treatment, his skin improved about 90 percent and the involvement of the disease in his bone marrow actually decreased. But while the interferon had its intended effect, it also had the usual and predictable side effects: flu-like symptoms, chills and fever, and a general and constant fatigue and malaise. In Rex's view, however, the side effects of interferon were certainly worth the benefits. He was alive, eating dinner almost every night with our family, teaching his priesthood and Sunday School classes every Sunday, actively serving as president of the nation's largest private university, running with me most mornings, and doing all the things that normal people do.

The other blessing we were given—and it was a rich one, indeed—was BYU. Instead of staying home and mourning another setback in Rex's health (and the obvious reality that his life would be shortened), he and I both worked. We did some of our work separately, as he put in his usual six days a week (plus many Sundays when he participated in religious activities that are integral to BYU). He attended to the many matters that find their way to the president's office, and he was the driving force behind many initiatives the university undertook. But we did much of the work together as we wrote talks, met with students, hosted dinners, traveled in the university's behalf, and immersed ourselves in the life of the university.

Perhaps the most memorable of many trips came soon after we received news of Rex's second cancer. It involved

traveling to Jerusalem, and as Rex attended countless meetings, I saw much of the land where our Savior had lived.

As I visited so many of the sites without Rex, my thoughts
instinctively turned to the fact that the life of Christ had been
filled with adversity but also with joy. Then, as Rex joined me
one day for a trip to the Sea of Galilee and on another day to
the Garden of Gethsemane, I realized that even though Jesus
had the power to walk upon the water, he also had the
strength to submit himself to the will of his father. These were
lessons I needed, given what I knew was ahead, and I returned
from the Holy Land grateful and renewed.

When we were home in Provo, we encouraged our children to join us in many of our university activities, particularly concerts, plays, art exhibits, and athletic events. They
also helped host dinners in our home, as had been the case
during our Washington years. Our lives were entirely centered
around BYU and our children, and we never tired of the job.
It was exhilarating, and we found that as we gave service to
the university, any pain we were experiencing dissolved. Our
involvement there activated our hopes, comforted our hearts,
and energized our spirits.

The opportunity to speak frequently was something I
enjoyed very much. The reading and writing I did in preparation for each address helped me focus my thinking, and as I
thought more deeply, I also began to feel more complete and
whole. Interestingly, as my identity became even more con-
nected to Rex's through our shared activities, I gained a
stronger sense of self, bringing us even closer together. Our
mutual respect likewise grew, and we saw ourselves as a team
as much in our individuality as in our togetherness. I had
spent my life as a wife, mother, and sometimes teacher, and
now I was his colleague.

Rex: As early as a few months after I returned to Provo from
Bethesda in 1987, I began to notice a slight tingling in my feet. It
didn't affect anything that I did, but it would not go away and

was a bit annoying. My oncologist in Provo, Dr. Bott, asked me if it felt as if I were wearing socks and gloves, and I told him those were the areas that appeared to be affected. He told me that the culprit was the drug vincristine, which had been part of my chemotherapy. What I was experiencing was a common side effect of that drug, he said, and although it probably would not get any worse, it probably would not get any better either. So I resolved to just live with the minor discomfort.

Toward the end of 1991, the tingling sensation, especially in my feet, led to a slight numbness, and my ability to maintain my balance was slightly impaired. In March 1992, Janet, my daughter Wendy, and I were just finishing up a five-mile run along the banks of the Provo River when, for no apparent reason, I stumbled and almost fell. This was the first time I had actually stumbled. From that time forward, my numbness and lack of balance slowly progressed. I remember another time in June 1992 when we were in San Diego for a Western Athletic Conference Presidents' Council meeting. I was running with Janet and three of our daughters. After a couple of miles, I simply was not able to run any more. I had to put my arm on Janet's shoulder for stability and walk back to our hotel. That summer my neurologist, Dr. Joe Watkins, ran some tests and concluded that what I had was peripheral neuropathy, a damage to the nerves in my peripheral nervous system that was affecting both my arms and my legs. He told me three things about peripheral neuropathy: first, he wasn't sure what caused it. It could have been the original cancer, the chemotherapy or radiation treatments, or the possibility that in attempting to cure my present cancer, my body's own mechanisms had misfired and damaged my peripheral nerves. Second, it could not be cured, and there was nothing that could be done to prevent its further progress. And third, he hoped that it would reach a "plateau" level and not progress any further, although he could not assure me that would happen.

All of these conclusions were confirmed that summer and fall by two specialists in both oncology and neurology, one at the University of Utah and the other, a colleague of Dr. Rosen, at

Northwestern. I saw Dr. Rozental at Northwestern for the first time in October 1992, right after the first BYU-Notre Dame game. (We lost that one, but we would get our revenge two years later in one of the sweetest events of my life. On that day, as on many others, I reflected on how grateful I was to be on this planet for such an occasion.) I asked Dr. Rozental at that time if there was any reason that I should stop running. He told me no but asked me to notify him if for any reason I was unable to run any more. I inferred (correctly, I believe) that he thought—though he didn't tell me—that that time would come.

In fact, it did come. I don't remember exactly when, but I remember that by the time of the June 1993 WAC Presidents' Council meeting, I was no longer running. It was not, of course, a matter of my legs all at once being unable to support more than a walk; it came on gradually. The pain, mostly in my legs, also increased gradually, and we sought the advice of medical experts who helped me deal with it in various ways.

Throughout this progression of events, I was grateful for the fact that neither my cancer nor my neuropathy affected my ability to carry out my responsibilities as president of BYU. The cancer was present, but its consequences were thus far undetectable. Some of the effects of the neuropathy were visible. I walked more slowly and sometimes had to stand in meetings to relieve the pain. At times my lack of stability was apparent. Because the neuropathy affects my hands, I had moderate difficulty with my handwriting, and I noticed it was more of a challenge than before to use a knife and fork, to button shirts, and to tie neckties. But none of these progressed beyond the category of "I wish it weren't so." Even with the cancer and the peripheral neuropathy, my work at BYU over these years continued unimpaired, with at least one notable exception.

During April 1993, my father was very ill, and Janet and I spent several days with him in Mesa, Arizona, where he was hospitalized. As I left his hospital room before returning to Provo, both he and I knew that we would never see each other again in this life. Yet right to the end of that visit, he maintained his sense of humor. As I was leaving his room, I received a phone call that lasted for several minutes. When I finally hung up, Dad asked me what it was about, and I told him we were having some problems in our athletic department, though nothing serious. A great fan of BYU, he responded, "Oh, that must be serious—far more serious than my impending death."

The following Saturday, my brother Doug called to tell me our father had passed away, and Janet and I began to make plans to drive to St. Johns, which is not accessible by commercial aircraft. When my friend Jon Huntsman learned of this news, he immediately called and insisted that my family and I make the trip on his airplane. He knew that my peripheral neuropathy made it extremely painful for me to travel long distances by car. I gratefully accepted.

During this time, I was experiencing an increasing swelling in my left leg, and by Monday it had become rather painful. My doctor ordered a sonogram, which revealed blood clots, and he immediately told me I would have to be hospitalized. I told him that was fine but that I could not remain in the hospital on Wednesday because I had to speak at my father's funeral. He made a comment about there being a double funeral if I left, and I soon realized that I was not going to be traveling to St. Johns.

Knowing this, I called Jon, told him of my circumstance, explained that we would not need the use of his plane, and thanked him for his generosity. He said, "Well, what about your family? Don't they plan to attend?" I responded that they did but that there was nothing wrong with their health and they would simply drive as we had originally planned. I resisted, but he insisted. Plans were made for my family to be flown to Arizona for the funeral.

Jon is generous with his means, but he also gives of his precious time. The next day, as I sat in my hospital bed working on an upcoming graduation talk, in walked Jon with Rick Majerus. Though Rick coaches basketball at BYU's in-state rival, the University of Utah, I have always appreciated that Jon introduced me to this man who has since become a very good friend.

He is best known for his coaching skills, and those who don't know him well see him as having a rather rough exterior. But the qualities of this man extend far beyond anything he has accomplished on the basketball court. As is the case with each of my friends, these two did much during their visit to lift my spirits during what turned out to be a rather lengthy hospitalization.

On Wednesday, as planned, my family flew to St. Johns, where Janet, with characteristic elegance, delivered the talk I had written. Then a week later, when my blood clots still had me confined to a hospital bed, she delivered my April commencement talk, demonstrating in a particularly public way that we did, indeed, perform my university job as a team.

Janet: Soon after we learned of Rex's peripheral neuropathy, I read a passage in *You Gotta Keep Dancin'*, a book by Tim Hansel, who had experienced a near-fatal climbing accident and had lived his life since in constant pain. "There is nothing wrong with happiness," he wrote. "It's wonderful. The only problem is that it's based on circumstances, and circumstances have a tendency to shift." Having experienced more than a few such shifts in our lives, I was intrigued by what he then said: "Joy, on the other hand, is something which defies circumstances" ([Colorado Springs: LifeJourney Books, 1985], p. 54).

For Rex and me, the only way we could survive was to adopt what we came to call "selective attitudes" and to make conscious decisions about how we would respond to the challenges we faced. On winter mornings, as my daughters and I jogged on a nearby indoor track, I became strangely drawn to the people there who would routinely run, walk, limp, or even push themselves in wheelchairs. Regardless of how we went about the task, we were each going to get around the track as best we could.

Then one morning as I rounded a curve, I saw two men walking together slowly. One was hooked up to an oxygen tank, while the other was pushing it for him. Each time they made it halfway around the track, they stopped for a minute as the man on oxygen regained his strength. My first impression was how wonderful it was that a man of such frail health would make the effort to come and walk the track. I could imagine the courage and determination that act required. Then, as I watched his companion, I realized that the example of each man was equally compelling. The courage of the one was admirable; the service of the other was Christlike.

That image serves as a great motivating force in my life as Rex goes through the changes that inevitably grow out of his condition. He has contracted countless infections as a result of his weakened immune system. We have learned to treat these with antibiotics, and he then invariably has gone to work, hoping the fever will subside. But the constant threat of infections makes life more of a struggle for him. I match my stride to his as his pace slows and as he begins to take stairs one at a time, instead of bounding up them two at a time as had always been his practice. I offer to help as he struggles to button his shirt each morning. I have yet to master the necktie.

I admire, love, and encourage him as he makes both conscious and unconscious decisions about living a full and productive and joyful life, despite his never-ending pain. I watch him grow in patience and empathy as he feels a unity with those who also hurt.

Rex: To be honest, as I faced the prospect of my second cancer, many of my thoughts did not coincide with what others have described as my typically optimistic mindset. My very first entry in my sixth bound journal was made at the end of that awful week in February 1990, and even though the news of my second cancer had by then taken a definite turn for the better, I still wondered as I wrote on that first page whether I would live to complete the new volume I held in my hands.

Four years and four months later, I did in fact fill the last page of that journal. The date of that last entry was July 3, 1994—seven years to the day from the time I was admitted to NIH. I looked back at that day in 1987 and realized that at that time, I had seen my chances of getting to 1994 as being about as good as Switzerland going to war. Life had moved at a rapid pace over the ensuing seven years, but I had moved right along with it—despite my second cancer and the peripheral neuropathy (as well as blood clots, surgery to repair a hernia, and finally having my wisdom teeth pulled just weeks before my fifty-sixth birthday).

July 3, 1994, also marked the fifth anniversary of the Monday I assumed my responsibilities as president of BYU. During those five years, I had worked with my colleagues in long-range planning for the university, in resolving numerous challenges that had come to us, in launching a capital campaign that we were confident would raise a quarter of a billion dollars for BYU, and in overseeing a period of construction on campus that rivaled the feverish pace of the Wilkinson era. I had watched as our football team upset the University of Miami, which was the number-one-ranked team in the country at the time; and I had traveled with BYU performing groups to Russia, eastern Europe, Spain, and the Middle East. I had hosted Ronald Reagan, former president of the United States (who at the end of his speech and question-answer period had regaled his audience with the latest jokes on the former Soviet Union, almost making me late for a flight I needed to catch to Washington, D.C.). I had also helped arrange for the visit of President George Bush during his presidential campaign in 1992. And Janet and I had attended the Heisman Trophy award ceremony for Ty Detmer.

In addition to all that went on at the university, I had argued nine cases before the United States Supreme Court (which was my idea of a hobby during my years as president) and had enjoyed a string of six straight wins even as my problems with peripheral neuropathy had worsened considerably.

More important than a fulfilling professional life was the extent to which I could still enjoy being with my family. Even with all the demands BYU placed upon me and Janet, we found opportunities for children to join us at various official functions;

we continued to take trips to Lake Powell as a family; and if we were in town, we always had everyone over for Sunday dinner.

I had been able to watch my son Michael leave on and return from his mission, and I had learned from him, among other things, that a "really cool" bike crash must involve, among other things, (1) at least half of the body ending up under the bike, (2) contact between the handlebars and either the chest or abdomen, and (3) at least some broken skin. (Foolishly, I had thought a bike crash was just a bike crash.)

There was no shortage of other momentous moments in our lives. On this day as I wrote, we were two weeks away from Stephanie's marriage to Bret Paulson. We had watched Michael marry Sharon Burr a year earlier. My signature was on the diplomas of Michael and Wendy, as well as four of our children-in-law, and Janet and I would watch with pride as Stephanie graduated a year later.

As I reached the five-year point in my presidency, I was well aware that I did have a very serious illness that would no doubt shorten my life. There were days of discouragement as I contemplated that reality. But I generally concluded that my best option was to be grateful for each day I lived and for a wife who helped to ensure there would be many more ahead.

I was also aware of the pain associated with my peripheral neuropathy. And while having to give up running was hard for me, I didn't have to reflect for long on what I sometimes viewed as my sorry state before I realized that there are millions of people in the world who live productive lives with much less mobility than that with which I have been blessed.

I spent a good deal of time writing on the third day of July. I expressed my gratitude to Janet, my Heavenly Father, and medical science for my blessing of life. I wondered what thoughts and events would fill my soon-to-be-started seventh volume. And I contemplated the words of one of my doctors when he said, "There are no peripheral nerves in the brain," which meant that even with decreased mobility I could do many of the things I enjoy in life.

My thoughts returned with some frequency to that statement. I began looking around at the way other people make their livings and realized how many depend so much on the use of their hands or their legs or both. I concluded that for about 85 percent of the working population in the United States, neuropathy at the stage mine had reached would mean unemployment. If I were a waiter in a restaurant or an automobile mechanic; if I had any of my old jobs on the sawmill; if I were an architect, dentist, almost any kind of physician; or if I made my living in so many other ways, I would be out of work—and would have been for several years. And given the way I am wired emotionally, forced unemployment would probably be about as difficult for me to take as my various physical ailments.

I also had this thought: Many people I know have much more serious physical problems than I, and many acquired these problems at a much earlier age. I repeatedly remind myself that for fifty-two years, I enjoyed almost perfect health. I literally cannot remember missing one day of work because of illness, though there may have been two or three when I should have. And these thoughts brought me back to my reaction that Friday in February 1990 when my friend Steve Freestone told me he and his partner had diagnosed my illness as mycosis fungoides: Every day is an extension of my life.

My final reflection as I filled that last page in my journal had to do with whether I would forgo what had happened and trade my circumstances at this point in my life for those eight years earlier, before my first cancer. There were obvious pros and cons, although I found it difficult to compare one category (what might have been) with the other (reality). The conclusion I came to that day was that yes, I would trade. But since the choice is not mine to make, I'll play with the cards I was dealt.

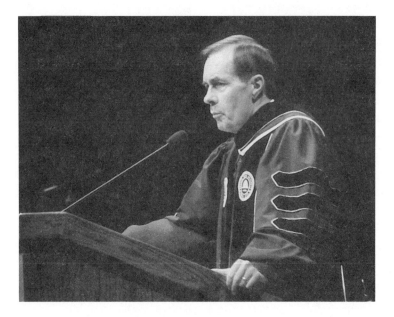

SOME OF REX'S FAVORITE MOMENTS AS PRESIDENT OF BYU WERE THE COMMENCEMENT EXERCISES HELD EACH APRIL AND AUGUST.

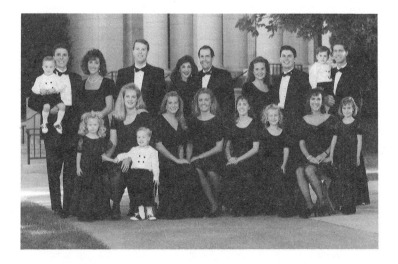

THE LEE FAMILY GATHERS IN FRONT OF THE KARL G. MAESER BUILDING AT BYU IN 1993.

CHAPTER 8

Pacing Ourselves

Rex: There were many things that helped to make the BYU presidency such a wonderful job. For me, probably the most prominent was the fact that unlike other responsibilities in the past, this was one that Janet and I truly shared. The law school deanship offered some opportunities in that respect, but not anything like being president. The other attractive features mostly had to do with relationships with people, the students, the faculty, the alumni and other friends of the university, and members of the board of trustees. Among the things that made it a challenge were the breadth of responsibilities and the inflexibility with which the work of that office must be carried out. In May 1995, I learned exactly what effect that inflexibility could have on me.

Thursday, May 4, came at the end of a very busy seven-day

period that had included our April commencement exercises, the ground breaking for our law school's new library, and a full slate of meetings with my president's council and the university's board of trustees. In a Thursday morning devotional assembly, Janet and I welcomed the participants of BYU's annual women's conference, and we then attended a luncheon for the organizers and special guests of that conference. After the luncheon, we went straight to the Salt Lake City airport and caught a three o'clock flight to the east coast, the principal purpose of which was to meet with some of our major donors, asking them to make large contributions to our capital campaign. I was feeling run-down as we headed out of town, but given the preceding week, that was no surprise.

In addition to our university business, we made a quick trip to Orlando, Florida, to see our daughter Wendy's new baby girl, Madeleine. We then spent Sunday in Washington, D.C., with our son Tom, who was living there with his family as he completed a Supreme Court clerkship. He and his wife, Kimberly, had a new baby boy, Bejamin Thomas, the fourth of four grandchildren born between January and April, starting with Michael and Sharon's twin boys, James Rex and John David. Janet and I had arranged our trip to be there for our newest grandson's blessing. Janet then stayed while I flew back to Utah for an important meeting on Monday morning, after which I was to return to Washington D.C., Monday evening. By the time I reached Provo Sunday night, I could feel one of my bacteria-induced fevers coming on.

For several years, I got one of these infections about every two months, sometimes more often. During my time at BYU, infections constituted one of my more serious and ongoing health challenges, though I had not yet recognized just how serious they could be. Infectious disease specialists had helped me during those years, and generally the best they were able to do was simply to treat the infections with antibiotics as soon as they began. Sometimes my temperatures would rise to 100 or 101, but my fevers were not accompanied by other symptoms of real illness. Usually, these temperatures would then subside in a matter of hours. But I could generally tell when the infection was serious. In those cases, my temperature would rise to something like 102 or 104, I would feel unusually weak, and I would develop serious chills at night.

All of those symptoms occurred Sunday night, and I started myself on an antibiotic the doctors had me keep on hand for such moments. The one problem with this antibiotic is that among the bacteria it destroys can be those that prevent yeast infections, which in some instances are even more serious than bacterial infections. As a consequence, whenever I took the antibiotic, I would accompany it with another drug that prevents yeast infections. One of the many things Janet helps me do is to keep track of my medications, and with her gone, I forgot to take the second drug with me as I packed Monday morning. (This was not the first time I had forgotten, and sometimes yeast infections would result and sometimes not.)

I would not have returned to Washington to complete the scheduled trip if I had felt I had a choice. I knew that my body, in its present condition, was simply not capable of meeting the physical demands that lay ahead. But I had no option. This trip had been planned for a month and a half, and two very busy and important people—Hyrum Smith and Dick Marriott—had scheduled time to be with me as we met with possible donors. All three of us, and also Tom Mullen, the BYU Development officer who accompanied us, were essential to the success of the trip, and Hyrum had scheduled his private jet to take us there. Those whom we were contacting had also set aside their time, and in several other respects the groundwork had been laid. After I had asked so many busy and important people to meet with me there was no way I was going to tell them that I didn't feel well enough to come.

Janet and I returned home Tuesday evening, and Wednesday I stayed home to rest (which, my secretaries later told me, was a sure sign that I was really sick). My temperature did go down considerably, and my general strength and feelings of well-being improved slightly. But then a yeast infection began to develop, and by Friday the inside of my mouth looked like a mature cotton field. I felt almost as sick as I had on Sunday night when I first started taking the antibiotic. There were several important things that I felt I had to do on Friday. The first was to meet with my dear friend Jon Huntsman, who gave me some of the best long-range advice I have ever received, and the last was to attend a wedding reception in Salt Lake. Janet had to drive us home, and I went right to bed. The next morning I felt as sick as I had in months, probably years, and my doctor told me to go to the hospital for some tests.

The doctors kept me in the hospital as they looked for the source of my infection, and I stayed in the hospital for sixteen days—my longest hospital stay in history, except for the four months at NIH. Doctors eventually located the source of the bacterial infection in my lungs, where they thought they also saw signs of cancer, including the original T-cell immunoblastic lymphoma that I had experienced in 1987. That possibility remained the principal diagnosis for several days, during which time surgeons entered my lungs from three different places to perform biopsies. They finally concluded that there had been no relapse of the immunoblastic lymphoma, although they found definite signs of the mycosis fungoides in my lungs. But as Dr. Rosen later said, he could have told them that without doing the biopsy. My present cancer is and always will be systemically spreading throughout my body, but it shows every sign of behaving itself.

Janet: Rex was very sick during these days of uncertainty, as the doctors ran a wide range of tests, came to various (sometimes conflicting) conclusions, and struggled to help my husband stay alive. Rex had been plagued with these recurring infections and fevers for over two years, but now nothing seemed to help him recover. He had always kept going when the infections came, but this time he was too weak to carry on in his typical routine of meeting with colleagues, dictating correspondence, and hosting visitors from his hospital bed.

From day to day, it took all his energy just to survive. We tried to keep visitors to a minimum because of Rex's sense that he needed to be up for friends who came to see him. Occasionally, when a custodian or lab technician would come into the room, Rex would come to life—asking where they were from, joking with them, and engaging them in lively conversations. But the children and I knew how ill Rex really was, and Christie commented one night that she was going to come the next day dressed as a custodian and carrying a mop so that she could enjoy him at his best.

I found it difficult to see him become weaker and weaker each day—this man who, when he couldn't run, had switched to a treadmill so that he could keep his balance as he continued to exercise; who, when he should have rested after his long days at work, attended every family event, helped children with homework, and made sure I always knew I was his very best friend. As the doctors looked for the source of the infection—and for signs of a spread of his cancer—Rex continued to grow weaker. He lost twenty-five pounds, and I wondered if this was to be the end.

Our daughter Melissa was in London for the summer attending BYU's Study Abroad program, and she and I were making long-distance arrangements for her wedding, which was scheduled for Friday, August 25. I wondered if I should have her come home early and whether we should go ahead with the wedding on schedule. When I asked Rex's oncologist, he was kind but frank. "Plan the wedding," he said, "and if Rex can be there, he will be there. If not, you're going to have to go on with your life."

This was a very matter-of-fact response to my heart's pleadings, and I wanted to scream, "We are discussing my husband—the love of my life!" Then, as I considered his response, I thought how hard I must be to please. On the one hand, I find it difficult responding to others' sad, pitying eyes and emotional voices. At the same time, it almost made me shudder to be met with such blunt objectivity.

As had been the case at NIH, it was difficult for me to leave Rex's room each night. Christie was our only child still living with us, and each night a friend would stay with her until I returned home. We would visit for a while, and then I would have some time to myself in the solitude of our home. I would read the thoughtful notes that friends had sent, water the plants, let the dog out, lock all the doors, and tidy up anything Christie and her friends hadn't cleaned up. I was actually glad for any little messes I could find, as they gave some sense of normalcy to the day. Then I would go through the nightly routine of getting ready for bed.

Most nights, sleep would elude me and my thoughts would match the blackness of the night. After praying and getting into our empty bed, I would return to my knees and continue to pray for Rex's recovery as well as for my own much-needed courage, calm, peace, and strength. I would reflect on scriptures I had read that day, on conversations with friends, on insights I had gained during our various challenges over the years. And I would try to remember a twofold lesson I have come to rely upon for strength: I am not alone, because my Heavenly Father is always with me; and I am not alone, because *everyone* faces such storms. They may come at different times, but we each will face our own difficulties and trials. They may come in different ways, but meeting those challenges and yet somehow finding peace seems to strike a universal chord in all of us.

As I struggled with my feelings during those dark nights, the thought of losing Rex wracked my soul. As I lay in our bed at home and thought about him at the hospital, I would try to turn my thoughts to the gratitude I felt—and wanted our children to feel—for the eight additional years we had been given with Rex. Eventually, I began to feel peace again. It was not a peace that freed me from concerns about Rex's condition or about the future; rather, it was a peace that came from feeling the strength of my Comforter. I was grateful I could recognize this power—and grateful for the many times I had felt it before.

For much of the time Rex was in the hospital, his condition was either worsening or barely staying level. When he had been at NIH, we had come up with the idea of trying to think of the most positive thing about each day as I prepared to leave; then I would try to focus on that during my trip home, even though much of the time I would just cry. (Some might view this trick as something of a delusion, but it seemed better than dwelling on the worst of what was happening.) We tried to do the same during this hospitalization, but there were several times when the best we could do, as we kissed each other good night, was to agree that tomorrow would be a better day.

On one particularly difficult day, my daughter Diana came and convinced me to go on a walk with her. While we were together, she asked how I could remain so calm and philosophical in the face of what was happening. I tried to explain to her that although my heart was breaking, I really had no other alternative—that, for me, falling apart and crying all day would only make matters worse. Through the difficulties Rex and I had faced over the years, I had come to realize that there are times when the only thing I can control is the way I respond to my circumstances. There are times when having dominion over my own attitude seems to be my sole means of exercising my God-given agency.

As Rex's condition continued to look bleak, our oldest son, Tom, came from Washington to be with his father. During Rex's good moments, the two of them discussed the law, a favorite subject for these two University of Chicago Law School alums. It was obvious that as Tom asked Rex his opinion on cases familiar to both them, Rex's spirits were lifted. Rex, however, was not the only one who was strengthened by Tom. When my son walked into the hospital for the first time and put his big arms around me, some of the burdens simply flowed from my consciousness. The memory of a little boy who had needed my hugs in exchange for his hurts was a million miles away, and it was now his turn to comfort me. In the days he spent with us, I felt that my burden was being lifted and carried by my son and that because of his assistance, I could relax a little. One night we returned home from the hospital and I started to take the trash bins out to the curb. Tom stopped me and took over. It was such a small act, but I began to cry as he headed out the door—and as I recognized the significance of his gesture and its effect on me.

Even after Rex was transferred out of the intensive care unit, he could walk only with the aid of two strong men—and then only for a few steps—before he was exhausted. It was during this time of "improvement" that Elders Neal A. Maxwell and Henry B. Eyring came to visit him, and I sensed that they were surprised at how ill Rex appeared. (Elder Maxwell was chairman of the executive committee of the board of trustees, and Elder Eyring was commissioner of Church education.) They stayed in the room for only a short time, and then the three of us spent a few minutes talking in the hall. They asked what they could do to help and then expressed the same thought I had been having—that somehow Rex was going to have to cut back on all he was doing.

Rex: My recollection of that hospital stay is hazy, at best. I do remember that I talked rather infrequently with my office and my vice presidents, that all of my children came to visit, and that I began hearing rumors that were circulating concerning the seriousness of my illness. Those reports irritated me, and I told Janet to tell people at BYU and in our ward that I was not as ill as had been reported. When I discovered after my release that, in this rare instance, the rumors had been correct—and that I had come very close to death—I began to wonder whether I could continue to keep the pace that was required of me at BYU.

The aftermath of that hospital sojourn was even more discouraging than the actual inpatient experience. For one thing, the days in the hospital were not my only "down time." Throughout my life I had been accustomed to bouncing back from illnesses rather quickly. Not so when I left the hospital in 1987, and not so when I left it on Memorial Day 1995. I was weak, lacking in energy, and simply unable to do the kind of work that my job demanded for more than a short period of time. To be sure, that circumstance improved, but the improvement was exasperatingly and uncharacteristically slow.

At the same time, my doctors, several of whom are also good personal friends, told me how serious this episode had been, that it had, indeed, been life-threatening, that it could happen again, and that I must make adjustments in my life to prevent its recurrence. They responded to my obvious question—"What should I do to prevent a recurrence?"—by emphasizing that I needed to avoid stress, long hours, and particularly inflexible demands that would not permit me to cut back when I felt an illness coming on. As I listened to each doctor describe things to avoid, I realized they were reciting my job description. Then I learned from Janet that one of my physicians, Dr. Tracy Hill (a pulmonary specialist who had become involved with my care during my bout with blood clots), had put the matter to her more directly when he asked, "Does he want to die in office?" In truth, I didn't; but the demands of my job and the fragile nature of my health simply were not compatible.

At the time I left the hospital, however, I was simply not emotionally prepared to resign. I had enjoyed my job too much and had programmed myself for several more years of similar activity. Janet was the first to bring up the possibility. I was lying on the couch resting, and I simply told her this wasn't the time to discuss the issue. But as the days went on, I pondered the matter myself and then did begin to discuss it with Janet. As much as I wanted my situation to be otherwise, it became very apparent that stepping down was the only option. It was not fair to my family, to me, or to the university to enhance the likelihood that something like this might happen again. To put it another way, I couldn't continue to have a job that lacked the flexibility to allow me to take steps as needed to prevent the recurrence of life-threatening illnesses.

On the first Wednesday of June, while I was in the midst of this agony, I attended the regular monthly meeting of the board of trustees, at which President Gordon B. Hinckley presided. At the conclusion of the meeting, President Hinckley asked to speak with me for a moment in his office. As we sat down, he said, "We're very concerned about you." The tone of his voice conveyed a compassion and genuine concern that adorn this great man so gracefully. In those simple words, which he repeated several times—"We're very concerned about you"—I felt an obvious outpouring of the prophet's concern. That brief conversation led me to conclude that the decision toward which I was leaning was the correct one. I acknowledged to him that in view of the fact that my health had taken a rather pronounced turn for the worse, I was concerned that I would not be able to continue as president of BYU, and he said he understood and then reiterated that his only concern was for my well-being. I asked if I could have his permission to meet personally with Elders Maxwell and Eyring and present a proposal which they could then approve or modify and present to him and the rest of the board.

On June 12, 1995, I met with Elders Maxwell and Eyring to discuss the matter. As I left for that meeting, Janet and I prayed, among other things, that Elder Maxwell would be inspired to advise us as to the best course to take. Prior to that prayer, I had not intended to include that request; I suspect the reason it came to me on that occasion was that I knew, from past association with him, of Elder Maxwell's deep compassion for other people and his similarly deep insights into what is best for them, especially in significant circumstances in their lives.

I began the meeting by reviewing for the two of them the circumstances that had led me very reluctantly, though quite clearly, to the conclusion that I should ask to be released. I then explained that because of several projects then under way at BYU, I felt the best time for my release would be in May 1996. I also reviewed three or four other personal requests that would help Janet and me make the transition back to teaching at the BYU law school and practicing law with the firm of Sidley & Austin.

As I concluded my thoughts, Elder Maxwell folded his hands, leaned back in his chair, paused for a few moments, and then said that he agreed with everything I had said and requested, with one exception: the timing of my leaving office. In his view, stretching my service out for another full year simply put too many demands and imposed too many risks on me. He suggested that a better time would be the end of the calendar year, which would give the board of trustees the opportunity to conduct a proper search for my successor.

I had two immediate reactions to this quite unexpected response. First, I worried about several projects that would be disrupted if I left at the end of the calendar year rather than the academic year. But Elder Maxwell had not taken those into account at all. They pertained to the interests of the university, and his only concern was for me. My second reaction was that though Elder Maxwell's counsel was not exactly what I expected, I had received exactly what I prayed for: his inspired judgment. As the three of us talked the matter through further, I saw adjustments that could be made to take care of, or at least diminish, all of the concerns I had.

The board of trustees approved my proposal on Friday morning, June 16, and that afternoon I announced my decision, together with my reasons for reaching the decision, to the entire BYU community. Their response at that meeting, which was held in the de Jong Concert Hall, will remain one of the outstanding memories of my life. I had been concerned that people might feel I was leaving prematurely, and without just cause, after six and a half years. There was no hint of that, either at the meeting or afterward. In fact, following the closing prayer I was surprised that there was a prolonged standing ovation, which I interpreted as an expression of love and appreciation.

Janet: Although we both knew the decision was right, making the request was one of the hardest things Rex had ever done. (Having him make the announcement was one of the hardest for me.) He did not want to fail the university in any way, and even though he eventually had to cut back somewhat on the time he spent in the office, he worked to keep his commitment to the BYU family that these last six months would be one of the most productive periods of his time in office.

As the two of us worked during these final months of his presidency, some of our friends suggested that Rex should reduce his workload, that his three hospitalizations in the intervening months indicated that he needed more rest than he was getting. I had similar thoughts at times, but I also knew that in Rex's case, being involved in something he loved was a great source of strength and possibly sustained him more than it impeded him.

I also heard comments at times questioning our way of dealing with Rex's cancer. Perhaps some people felt that by attempting to preserve some degree of normalcy in our lives, we were denying our inevitable mortal separation. It is true that neither one of us felt inclined to dwell on that eventuality. Once, as Rex and I were leaving one of our many doctors' appointments, the doctor suggested that we ought to take some time to discuss death and dying. As we drove away, I asked Rex if that was something he thought we should talk about. He weighed the option very quickly and said, "No, let's talk about living. I'm hungry, so why don't we go get a burrito before the basketball game." What is also true, however, is that underneath the routine of our very busy lives was the constant heartache of accepting that we would not grow old together, as we had always dreamed of doing. Though our innermost feelings remained unseen by others, the reality of Rex's condition followed us like our shadows—which are their smallest when the sun is the highest. But reality, like shadows, often loomed larger than either of us could bear for more than a few moments at a time.

Rather than dwelling unduly upon such thoughts, however, we smiled, we laughed, and sometimes we cried; then we went about our lives as "normal" people do. We tried to see life with all of its goodness and beauty and ourselves as part of this glorious world. I often thought that I did not want to spend my time looking through a periscope of fear, where all I could see would be an ocean of black. If I focused only on Rex's poor health, on the things he no longer could do, and on my eventual loss, I would not be able to see and enjoy all that we still share together. Nor could I deny the miracle of enjoying life together eight and one-half years after his first cancer was diagnosed.

Two events in our family's lives bridged the weeks between the end of BYU's 1995 summer term and what we now knew would be our last semester on campus. First, our daughter Stephanie graduated—the last of three of our children whose diplomas bear Rex's signature. When Rex first became president, Stephanie was sixteen and had reservations concerning his new position. In her mind, having a father who was also president of BYU brought embarrassing attention to her and her family. But as she walked across the stage on this August day and received not only her diploma but a hug and a kiss from the university's president, she viewed his role at BYU very differently than she had six years earlier. And when she took her seat and was asked by some fellow students why she rated a kiss from the president, she proudly declared, "He's my dad."

Two weeks later, our daughter Melissa was married to Brett Wimmer, the son of our friends from many years before, Larry and Louise Wimmer. At their wedding luncheon, Rex was his usual charming and jovial self as he made a few remarks as the father of the bride. But he also reflected with tenderness on his eternal perspectives of birth, marriage, children, and death, and his remarks had particular meaning to all who were there. I often thought about the fact that Melissa and Brett had met quite by chance; but Brett, having experienced the loss of his own mother to cancer several years before, was able to provide a unique form of support to

Melissa, who was having to deal with her father's weakening condition.

Just before Thanksgiving of 1995, Rex spent several days in the hospital as the doctors tried once again to get his pneumonia under control. Rex's body responds better to intravenous antibiotics than oral ones, so it was decided to insert a Hickman catheter into his chest, which would also provide a central line for any other intravenous procedures he needed. As I contemplated administering the antibiotics when we returned home, I thought back to the many medical procedures I had learned to deal with over the years—giving shots, changing dressings, determining which ointment would soothe his raw skin, checking for swollen lymph nodes, and watching for the hollow eyes that let me know Rex was pushing himself beyond reason.

During these days, I would sometimes think back to the fact that even as a little girl, I had never wanted to be a nurse. I used to feel faint at the mere smell of the alcohol doctors use to cleanse wounds. Yet here I was, immersed in Rex's care and unable and unwilling to turn my back on what had become the heartbeat of my life. The once-unfamiliar CAT scan rooms, treatment procedures, and hospital stays were becoming familiar to me; and at the same time I was coming to appreciate how good it feels to be free of pain, because I could see how terrible it is to suffer from it.

Perhaps exceeded only by the experiences of birth and death, pain is one of the experiences most common to all of humanity. Even the Savior, in his perfection, was not free from it. In my own way I was learning the relationship between suffering and happiness, and that my awareness of joy was not found in freedom from torment but through finding peace in its midst.

I knew that much of the peace both Rex and I enjoyed came directly from our Heavenly Father and that some came from those sent in his behalf. I came to regard the nurses and other hospital staff who cared for Rex—and, in less visible ways, for me—as angels of mercy. The doctors in charge of his constant care (whose numbers make naming each one impossible) exercised judgment I often sensed was inspired, and they became close friends. Our neighbors and friends far and wide offered many outward expressions of support, as well as their less visible love, concern, and prayers. My father and mother, who live in Provo, helped our children and grandchildren with things I would ordinarily do, and Rex's mother would call frequently from Arizona and would lift Rex's and my spirits each time she did. Rex's brothers and their wives—Doug and Dixie, Richard and Clarice, and Mark and Robin—offered love and support in ways that only family members can give. My brother Glen, a doctor himself, and his wife, Mary Ella, a nurse gave comfort to both our bodies and souls. My sister Lois and her second husband, Alan, warmed our hearts in ways that few can. Our children, likewise, supported by our four sons-in-law and two daughters-in law, would often turn the tables by providing for our needs. Somehow each one knew exactly what to do and say at precisely the time things needed to be said and done. The years of sharing encircled us with love.

Even with the support of so many, I often thought about something my mother shared with me long before Rex's first cancer. She said that when I was young, she would always give me plenty of warning before bedtime or any other intrusion into my activities, because then I could meet the change cheerfully. Through all of our challenges over the ensuing years, I have seen how well my Heavenly Father knows me and how he shows his love as a parent by giving me some sort of warning and then time to prepare. With my husband once again in the hospital, I couldn't help but think of the greatest challenge that I knew Rex and I were yet to face, but I was grateful that my Heavenly Father was allowing me time to prepare for what was ahead.

When Thanksgiving Day came, we spent much of our time in the usual preparations for our meal together. Six of our seven children were with us, together with five in-laws and eight grandchildren, which made for a very busy day. In the middle of all the preparations, however, my mind kept returning to our Thanksgiving eight years earlier, just after Rex had returned from NIH. On that day, we were frightened, sad, and almost hesitant to be grateful because of our inability to see what was ahead for Rex. If I had known then that in 1995 I would be spending yet another Thanksgiving with Rex, and if I could have seen the extent of our joy over these eight years together, I could not have contained my joy.

As we sat down to eat, I admired the table and the food, but I knew that what I was really enjoying was the spirit that was in our home. As we took turns expressing our individual thanks, I marveled that each person momentarily forgot the physical trappings that sometimes can seem so important in our lives and concentrated instead on our family's eternal blessings. When Rex took his turn, he spoke specifically of each of our seven children, our six children-in-law, and our ten grandchildren, expressing, as he did so often, how proud he was of each of their unique talents and abilities. He and I then expressed our appreciation for each other and for a kind and loving Heavenly Father who had allowed us this extra time together to be with our children and grandchildren. I noticed a few well-concealed tears around the table, but I knew they were not tears of sorrow.

Later that night, I continued to reflect on what our life had been like eight years earlier and what it was like in 1995. I remembered how I had thought, upon getting out of bed that dreadful morning in Boise, that the carefree joy of youth had been taken away from me and that I would never be the same again. I have learned to understand that I was only partially right. That naive happiness has given way to something of far greater substance—a deeper joy that I could never have known without the challenges of the intervening eight years.

In that time, Rex and I have loved life to the fullest. We have shared laughter and optimism, as well as silent struggles and efforts to be strong. We have prayed separately and together, shedding tears, composing ourselves, and then entering our world once again with happy hearts. Time and time again, we have been shown how quickly despair can turn into delight as we have enjoyed the world and all that is in it.

There are so many things we have learned over these eight years. But as I thought through them over and over before I went to bed that Thanksgiving night, I knew that the most important lesson for me was the realization that I will always be happy—that no matter what happens in a future that neither Rex nor I can clearly see, no matter how dark the night becomes before the sun rises again, I will always know joy.

Rex: As the end of 1995 approached, I was concerned that I spend my last weeks as president of BYU as productively as possible. There were many matters that still required my attention. My health, however, was not cooperating in the way I had hoped. While I did spend much of my time at the university, I also worked from a hospital bed during two different stays in the months of November and December. The second hospitalization was the week before Christmas, and there was some concern that I wouldn't be released before December 25. Two days before Christmas I had improved sufficiently to be home for Christmas with Janet and every one of our children, including their husbands and wives, and all ten of our grandchildren.

Janet's and my Christmas gift to our children and their spouses that year was a vacation we were scheduled to take together on January 3, and there were understandable concerns about whether I would be able to make that trip or not. Janet, in particular, was worried that it might be hard for me not to be able to join in all the activities. But my thought was that even with my limitations, I could still enjoy being with my fourteen favorite people in this world, and I could participate in their activities vicariously.

As I packed up my office at BYU, I was not without emotion, but as I left and knew that the office would be occupied by my dear friend Merrill Bateman, I was excited about the prospects of returning to the practice of law, teaching at the law school, and trying to get a little more rest, which everyone told me I needed.

During the first two days of our one-week vacation, I felt better than I had in months. My neuropathy made it difficult for me to get around, but I had brought work with me, and I really did enjoy relaxing, working some, and watching our family enjoy themselves. The second day, as Janet worried about leaving me alone while she and the children went on a hike along a trail she and I had discovered together sixteen years earlier, I told her, "I'm as happy as a clam," which pretty well summed up my state of mind at that moment.

Janet: Before the children and I returned from our hike, Rex knew he was getting sick, and by that evening he had developed a fever. We contemplated cutting the trip short, which Rex wouldn't hear of; so after consulting with our doctor in Provo, I started him on the intravenous antibiotics we had packed but had hoped we would not have to use. Fortunately, within twenty-four hours his fever did subside even though he was still very weak. We all tried to keep him comfortable as he encouraged us to get out, have fun, and then share our experiences with him.

The flight home can only be described as miserable, and it was evident by the time we landed in Salt Lake City that Rex needed to return to the hospital. He insisted that we go home first, largely so that the children wouldn't be overly concerned about his condition, but we were there only a few minutes before we knew he could not stay.

As had been the case for so many years, my foremost concern was Rex's health, while his was the work he had to do and the commitments he had made. In particular, he was concerned with being able to make an upcoming trip to Denver, Colorado, where he was scheduled to argue a case in behalf of BYU before the U.S. Court of Appeals for the Tenth Circuit on

January 25, 1996. And, as had generally been the case, he did respond to the antibiotics and was able to leave the hospital a week later. This time, however, he left with an oxygen tank that now helped supplement the needs of his ailing lungs.

Before leaving on Rex's trip to Colorado, we found ourselves growing more comfortable with our new routine, which involved monitoring oxygen levels, administering antibiotics through Rex's Hickman catheter, and providing respiratory therapy, but which also involved enjoying the many things we *were* able to do. Through it all, Rex remained remarkably active, driving himself to meetings and climbing stairs when he probably should have taken elevators.

One day, Rex was able to walk into the law school to hear our son Michael argue in the annual moot court competition. Rex was overcome with emotion to even be there, and when Michael took first place, he enjoyed a moment of understandable pride. When we left for Denver a short time later, however, Rex was feeling quite weak, and so we rented a wheelchair for him to use on the trip. Pushing him through the two airports while juggling his oxygen tank was a new experience for me, but by the time we reached the courthouse in Denver it had almost become second nature. When I hit a bump and almost knocked him onto the floor, Rex continued to joke with the other lawyers, asked me to turn his oxygen up, and rearranged the papers that had slipped from his lap— all in a casual manner that distracted us from the fact that this was the first time he had entered a courtroom in a wheelchair and on oxygen.

For a moment, as he approached the bench to plead his case, it was sobering to see him looking frail and sitting in a wheelchair instead of standing tall as I had seen him so many times before. But as his confident voice began, "May it please the Court . . . " I saw how glad he was to be there. We were where he wanted to be, he was doing what he loved and did so well, and there was no space for sadness.

When his argument was over, we returned to the courthouse halls, greeted friends, briefly discussed the case with the other BYU lawyers, and then braved the cold Denver winter on our short walk back to our hotel for lunch. We found a table convenient for a wheelchair, checked Rex's oxygen level, and ordered soup and salad. Rex was jubilant, the conversation was lively, and I found myself forgetting our new circumstances. Rex wanted things to be normal, and as nearly as possible, we made that happen.

We returned to Provo later that day, and as Rex fell asleep that night, I reflected on one of our first days at NIH, when I talked briefly with a woman who was pushing her husband through the hospital halls in a wheelchair. When she told me he had been battling cancer for ten years, I didn't think I could ever do what she was doing, but my time had come and I found I could. Now, almost nine years later, I bowed my head and thanked my Father in Heaven for giving me the strength to do what I had to do. As I offered that quiet prayer, however, I felt gratitude for something more than strength: I felt joy and peace as I thought about helping Rex do all the things he loved doing. We still laughed and talked and prayed together. I still liked us.

Rex awoke and found me with damp eyes. "What's with you?" he asked. "I'm just happy," I answered honestly, and he squeezed my hand.

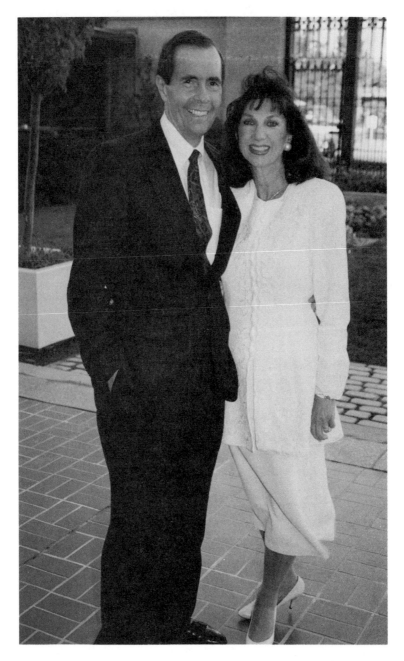

REX AND JANET AT TEMPLE SQUARE IN SALT LAKE CITY, UTAH

CHAPTER 9

Reflections

Rex: If I could trade my physical body of 1995 for the body I had in 1985—even allowing for the normal deterioration that comes with age—I would surely do so. Nevertheless, I have learned some valuable lessons, and as those lessons have been added to my fund of knowledge and understanding, my life has improved correspondingly. Inevitably, we learn from any of life's experiences.

This is not to say that I recommend cancer, chemotherapy, and peripheral neuropathy as a way of improving your life. I don't; the costs are far too high. But I think it is possible for other people to learn these same lessons vicariously without having to endure the difficulties others have experienced. What I've learned may also be helpful for people who have the same or similar health challenges as I do. For both groups I offer the following thoughts.

Probably the most important thing I have learned is the value of life. I clearly recognize how essential it is to appreciate life and the many blessings it offers—not just as we look back in retrospect, but right now, at the very moment that the good things in life are happening to us. Prior to 1987, I had never given these matters any thought. Life was just there, and I lived it. Days, weeks, and months passed, and months in turn evolved into years, each year seeming to go by a little faster than the previous one. But I never gave any thought to the reality—or the consequences of the reality—that this succession of mortal time segments would not go on forever. Just as we assume that cancer is something that happens to someone else, so also we often feel that the end of mortality lies in such a distant future that there is no point in thinking about it.

And then, on June 22, 1987, I suddenly and abruptly faced the probability that I would never experience 1988, and I of course immediately began to long for more time. When my cancer was later declared to be in remission and I was released from the hospital and returned to a more normal life in Provo, I had an entirely different outlook on life and the segments of time of which life, after all, consists. Every day, every week, every year was a bonus. I felt that way in 1987, and I have felt that way ever since.

The point was brought home to me again in February 1990, when for three horrible days—probably the worst days of my life—I once again thought I would never see another Christmas, probably not even the upcoming BYU graduation in April. Then, when I was told that I had a less aggressive form of cancer than the initial diagnosis had indicated and that I could live for somewhere between three and thirteen more years, I was literally ecstatic. My mind raced through all the wonderful things that could happen to me even if I were granted only three additional years. In my relief, I felt it was not that my life had been shortened; rather, it had been extended.

I concede that because of my illnesses it is probably easier for me than for most people to regard each passing day as a bonus, but there is no logical reason that others who have not had a life-threatening disease cannot learn from my experience rather than having to endure it themselves. We can learn to appreciate the value of each of the days, months, years, or decades to which we look forward.

The second lesson I learned centers around the same issue of appreciating the value of life and health—not from the standpoint of the "here and the now" or the future, but rather in retrospect. Since the time of my illnesses, I have noticed many people, both friends and strangers, whose physical abilities have been impaired, many of them much more seriously than mine and at a much younger age. I am now deeply grateful for the fact that I had fifty-two years of virtually perfect health, with hardly a day of sickness during all that time. During those fifty-two years, my energy supply was virtually inexhaustible. I was able to run thirteen marathons, including two at Boston and one that I finished in under three hours. Today, my energy supply is very definitely exhaustible. Not only am I unable to run marathons; I cannot run at all. But I appreciate in retrospect those fifty-two good years.

A closely related fact is that I can still do much that makes my life happy. To be sure, there are a lot of things I can't do— things I see my friends doing, things in which I wish I could participate. One of the things I have learned in this respect is that attitude, mind-set if you will, is all-important. Just as it is crucial for me to regard life as having been extended rather than shortened, it is equally important to concentrate not on the things that I cannot do but on things that I still can do that can make my life very happy if I will let them.

This latter effort has at times been difficult, because I have struggled with two conflicting inner voices. Each of them speaks to me on a regular basis. My conflict is, to which of these should I listen? The first says, "Isn't it a shame? You'll never run another marathon. To put it bluntly, you have become to the marathon what Bart Simpson is to the Nobel Prize. You remember all those roughhouse games you used to play with your children, and how many pleasant memories you associate with them? How much of that can you still do? And remember that week-long hike you took with your son Tom and other Boy Scouts into the Uintahs, and you'd always planned to take that hike again with the entire family? Well, forget it. And what about Lake Powell? It will never be the same again. Cliff jumping and water skiing are out of the question. So are the long hikes that include climbing steep sandstone hills. Things are really bad."

The other voice says, "Things are really good. You are alive. Because your central nervous system is unaffected by your illnesses, you can still engage in challenging and interesting intellectual activities. There are still games you can play with your grandchildren, including many of the same ones you used to play with your children. And Lake Powell? You can drive the boat, ride on the water weenie, and laugh and joke and play with your children and grandchildren. Come to think of it, it isn't all that bad to be the one who stands on the bow of the boat and yells out instructions as to where to put the anchors. What you now have is a legitimate excuse to pick the cushy jobs and leave the tough ones to someone else."

I faced a similar conflict when I came out of the hospital in May of 1995. The experience left me very weak and lacking in energy. Regaining that energy was exasperatingly slow and initially was the cause of considerable discouragement and even a bit of resentment. To be sure, my energy was increasing, but the rate of increase was tortoise-like. What I found was that I had to concentrate not on comparing my energy level with what it had been before I went into the hospital but with what it had been the week before.

After my cancer was diagnosed, a topic of conversation that was difficult to discuss centered around the reasons I may have gotten cancer and the reasons I was later cured. Some wanted to discuss the question "Why me?" I think that included within that simple little two-word question are two elements. The first is the question "Why was I the one who got cancer?" That question, interestingly enough, was never one I asked myself. But many of my friends did ask it, some of them with a tinge of resentment and some with more than just a tinge. The second element of the question is "Why did I survive, when others— people who were every bit as worthy, every bit as needed by their families, and for whom just as many family members and friends prayed just as fervently—are not alive today?" That second question is the one I asked.

With regard to the first question, the question of why I got cancer, Janet and I heard comments based on two quite opposite premises. The first and probably the most common idea was that bad things—or at least really terrible things like cancer—just shouldn't happen to good people. That is a notion with very ancient roots.

Consider Job. His friends felt that his terrible illnesses were a manifestation of his wickedness. Some of our acquaintances seemed to wonder the same things Job's friends wondered: What had I done to deserve this illness? I often thought, when that question was raised, of a similar question put to the Savior concerning a blind man: "Who did sin, this man, or his parents, that he was born blind?" (John 9:2–3).

During my stay at NIH, I received a card from a longtime friend at the Justice Department with whom I have carried on a longstanding and good-natured banter about the net value of my Mormon lifestyle. His card contained a six-word variation on this theme that has prevailed from Job's day to ours. His card said, "Well, so much for clean living."

The other assumption, made by some other friends and acquaintances, was quite the opposite from the first: In their view, my cancer was due to my righteousness, rather than the lack thereof. I was being tested because I was so valiant.

This response reminded me of a story I've heard Elder Dallin H. Oaks tell about the man who was being ridden out of town on a rail and who commented that if it weren't for the honor of the thing, he would just as soon walk.

For me, the answer to the first aspect of the "Why me?" question seems fairly clear. I got cancer not because I was particularly wicked or because I was particularly righteous. The Savior himself made that clear in his answer to the question about the blind man. The Savior explained, "Neither hath this man sinned, nor his parents: but that the works of God should be made manifest in him" (John 9:3). I believe that what this and other scriptures teach is that the plan under which we are here necessarily assumes that we are on our own as to many matters, and one of those is susceptibility to serious illness or other disasters. If our Heavenly Father intervened to spare really good people from those kinds of experiences, much of the effect of this life's developmental and testing process would be blunted. If it were readily and objectively determinable that living a certain kind of life—either good or evil—in effect immunized a person from many of life's crises, it would be much easier to persuade people to live such a life. As it is, the case must be made exclusively on the merits of living a good life.

What about the second question, the one I asked myself: Why have I been spared, when others with similar illnesses have died? Here again, my friends—this time by the trainload—have been willing to supply the answer. My life was preserved, they say, because there were important things for me to do here—specifically, my work as president of BYU since 1989. I think that is what Janet believes in her heart.

I respect that view, and I acknowledge that it may be correct. But I am reluctant to accept it unequivocally for three reasons. First, it seems inappropriate and immodest for me to take that view when, in fact, other sons and daughters of God have such important missions to fulfill on earth. Second, every argument—and I mean *every* argument, including the one that the Lord needed a BYU president to succeed Jeff Holland—that could be made as to why I have been left on this earth can also be made for my friend Terry Crapo, whose cancer took his life in 1982, and to others as well. Certainly someone else could have served in my place. And finally, the only thing that is really certain is that we just don't know why some people recover from serious illness while others, with the same illness, the same worthiness, and the same faith and prayers, do not.

Both the scriptures and my own personal experiences and observations make it very clear that formal, extraordinary efforts (principally fasting and prayer) to invoke divine intervention on behalf of loved ones are proper, should be undertaken, and frequently bear fruit. But we cannot be assured this will always be the case. Indeed, if it were the case, two of the fundamental premises of this existence—the need for independent earthly experiences and the need to be tested—would be frustrated.

Far more important to me than knowing why I recovered from the first cancer and why the second has been kept at bay is taking full advantage of the fact that both things have happened, in fulfillment of the most fervent prayers that I have ever offered. What I do know is that I am alive; I am able to live outside a hospital, away from an IV pole, and to do work that I love; and I am blessed with a family whom I love and particularly with a wife who during so many difficult times gave me a new insight into what love really means.

The Savior has told us that we should love one another even as ourselves. I take that quite literally as the ultimate manifestation of love: concern and feeling for every other human being. Christ himself is the only person who has achieved that state. But during my many illnesses, I learned that it is possible to achieve that complete love for some individual people. And I saw it in Janet toward me. I came to realize, quite literally, that my life, my welfare and happiness, were just as important to her as were her own.

I first saw it manifest in her decision to go with me to NIH. On its face, that seemed like quite an impractical decision, even bordering on irrationality. We had a large family, all of whom needed caring for and four of whom were still living at home. And the youngest was just a small child. It made little sense for her to leave these responsibilities and travel two thousand miles east to be with me when, as I assumed at the time, there was little she could do since she was not a doctor. But I could soon tell that this was not an open issue; she was going. And she did.

The depth of her feelings for me became even more apparent once we arrived in Bethesda. I deeply appreciated her direct involvement with the doctors, her in-depth acquisition of understanding about the nature of my disease and its possible treatments, and her voluntary involvement as part of my medical team. Any one of the doctors was with me, at the most, once or twice a day, usually for less than a half hour. But Janet was there virtually all the time. She saw things they did not, simply because she was a more constant observer. And because she had at least a good working knowledge of some of the characteristics of my cancer, and because her instincts for health matters are borderline phenomenal, she could pick up signals that they did not. Time after time at NIH and in the years since then, she would make suggestions as to things that ought to be done—and she was not at all hesitant to make them. The doctors and nurses soon came to respect her ideas because more often than not they had real merit.

To be sure, she was not at the hospital every hour of every day, but she was there most of the time. And I began to worry about her health—her emotional if not her physical health—when I considered the amount of time she spent at the hospital. We had many friends in the area because for five of the preceding six years, the Washington, D.C., area had been our home. These friends noticed Janet's constant attention to me and were concerned about the same thing as I. They would go out of their way to invite her to events that might take her mind, at least temporarily, away from my illness. Consistently, I would urge her to accept those invitations or at least to do something that would take her outside the hospital. I was always telling her, "Look, I have to stay here. I have no choice. But you do. I appreciate your being here, but you shouldn't have to bear this much of my burden." And in fact, she did accept a few of those invitations, principally to accommodate people whose only objective was to be helpful. But she always said that during those times her mind was focused mostly on what might be happening in my hospital room.

These acts of love were not limited to Janet. Each of our children—at many different times and in many different ways—have demonstrated their love for me and helped me endure the challenges I have faced.

When I left Provo to travel to NIH in June of 1987, I was facing the probability that I would never see another Christmas with my family. When my second cancer was initially diagnosed in February 1990, I felt certain that I would not see my son Michael leave on his mission (let alone return), would not witness any more of my children being married or graduating from high school or college, and would not do many of the other things that fill parents with joy. I have no idea why I have lived for so many years beyond what anyone expected. What I do know is that I have savored and will yet savor every moment I spend with a wife and children who have, through their love, made each day of my life worth living.

Janet: It is a wet winter morning near the end of 1995. I have awakened especially early and have decided to head out for a run by myself, despite the dark, cloudy sky and the fact that I will have to run alone. Usually, I much prefer to run with Diana and Melissa, but we didn't made arrangements last night and it is too early to call.

I dress quietly, so as not to disturb Rex, and go downstairs to let the dog out while I finish tying my shoes. Before I even have my second shoe tied, Ike is scratching at the door, begging to come back in and thus alerting me to the fact that it is cold and rainy. For a second, I consider running on Rex's treadmill, but I decide the time in the quiet outside will be worth getting drenched. So I step out into the cool morning, closing the door behind me. As I run down our driveway and head south toward the Provo Temple, I feel free and happy to be outside. As I pick up speed and dodge a few puddles, I think about what it means to close a door and move ahead once a decision is made.

My feet move at a steady pace, and I think of the marathon I ran in 1994 with Diana, Wendy, and Stephanie. When I began training for this race, I could barely comprehend running 26.2 miles. I had been running six miles a day for years, but the thought of running more than four times that distance seemed impossible. But with incremental increases, I soon found that running twelve miles seemed more effortless to me than running five miles had years before.

The marathon itself was harder than I had imagined, particularly the last seven miles. I found myself trying to look ahead, wondering what hills I had yet to climb. I also looked back, worrying about who might be passing me. Whichever way I looked, my pace seemed to slow. Then, as is common in marathons, another runner joined me and said, as if he could read my mind, "Don't get discouraged . . . I've run this race before. The end isn't as bad as it may seem from here, and there's water up ahead." Then he went on.

I think about how difficult it would be for me to keep running through the cold if I kept looking back at the door or too far ahead in anticipation of my destination. I wouldn't notice the sky as it begins to lighten, smell breakfast cooking at a neighbor's house, or see white ribbons of smoke drifting from another's chimney. It makes me feel warm, in the chill of the morning, to be among neighbors who are awakening to the beginning of a new day.

My route through our neighborhood is a nice change from my usual run up Provo Canyon. When I head up the canyon, somehow I have the sense of running away from my cares. This morning, I feel more centered, more grounded to my world of reality. There is no conversation with my daughters; I am left simply with my own thoughts. As I pass the temple and run down the hill toward the Missionary Training Center, I can tell that this is going to be a soul-searching morning. I feel a sense of contentment and peace, and I know this will be a good run. I haven't been able to run in a few days, so it feels especially good to have the wind in my face and hair as I slip deeper into my thoughts.

My mind turns to the many times Rex and I ran this route together. We ran it in the fall, when leaves crunched beneath our feet. We ran it in the winter, with snow dusting our faces. Together we marveled at the new birth of springtime, and in summers we felt the scorching sun. What a wonderful cycle the seasons make, and we have enjoyed them all.

I think of Rex at home, still sleeping. Last night as I was falling asleep with my head on his shoulder, I listened to the rhythm of his breathing. I had just finished giving him a ten-day cycle of intravenous antibiotics, and the whistling and wheezing were gone from his lungs. My memory of those clear, deep breaths is like a song in my ears and makes me smile. Our past experiences tell me that the pneumonia will return, possibly within a few days, and I know I must enjoy each day that he is free of infection.

I think of him awaking, and I wonder if that simple act each day is like a bad dream for him as his senses surface, his pain registers more keenly, and he is once again aware of all he cannot do.

When he awakes, he will know where I am. At first, when he couldn't run, I felt I should stay home too, but he insisted, with his characteristic unselfishness, that I go ahead without him. "There's no point in both of us staying here," he would tell me. He is always logical, but still I would feel guilty as I left the house. For a time, I would walk with him and then run either before or after that time together. But the neuropathy has advanced now to the point where even walking to his car is an effort.

Seeing Rex in pain is hard for me. He tells me that it never ceases. There is effort in his breathing. His legs ache and are getting harder to move all the time. Yet I am learning that it doesn't help either of us if I allow myself to feel his discomfort so personally that I become his partner in pain. What he needs more than my empathy is my strength.

We are dealing with changes in our lives. Rex's care takes much of my time, yet I now find tasks routine that a few years ago I could not have imagined performing. As we take one day at a time, we are adjusting to new treatments, new medications, and new needs. I now must button Rex's shirts, and I help him up and down the stairs. Recently, in an uncharacteristic moment of frustration, he said to me, "I'm no good to you anymore. I just can't do what I used to be able to do for you." I assured Rex that he remains everything he has ever been to me, that I know what he is and what he will always be, that I really do not see him as any less than what he has always been. It was typical of him that within a few minutes, he was able to set the frustration aside and move on with the day.

Continuing on with our happy lives is important to both of us. Although we are constantly reminded of the progression of his illness, we never give up hoping for more time together. I remember that a few days ago, a doctor said something that made my heart glad. I had asked him how long a particular treatment Rex was receiving would last, and he responded that it could go on for years. I didn't question him. I elected instead to be left with the thought that the two of us could be together for years to come.

As I turn north and run along Timpview Drive, I look up at Mount Timpanogos, which is shrouded in a thick white cloud that dwarfs her majesty. A blanket of snow will cover her for several more months, and storms will blow against her surface. But neither wind nor rain nor snow will wear her down. The vegetation will lie dormant under her cold, white crust, but with the warmth of spring will come rivers and streams, nourishing the flowers and greenery that will come alive again and delight the strong and brave who are determined to reach new heights. But until spring, Timp will undergo a much-needed metamorphosis, as her ground soaks up the moisture it will need to produce life once again. I wonder if I, too, am in a time of preparation and nourishment that will help me stand against greater storms to come.

We have been through such a mixture of seasons, Rex and I. One day it is winter, then the next day it's spring. It all depends on how he feels or what a doctor says. Some days, we feel the winds of winter for an hour, and then spring bursts forth as we attend a dinner, a devotional, a musical, or a sporting event. Our spirits soar and then they slide, but through the ups and downs we feel a gentle peace that all is well, that God *is* in his heaven, and that he is aware we are here. We feel comfort knowing that he whose will shall be done knows us and loves us.

I run as far north as Timpview Drive goes and then turn south again on my way home. I want to be home for a few minutes with Christie before she leaves for school, and I need to help Rex get ready for the day. As I run past Rock Canyon School, where each of our seven children attended elementary school, I watch three children dart across the crosswalk, with lunchboxes held tightly and backpacks hanging like camels' humps over their bulky coats. In my mind's eye, I see my own children as they were a few years ago: Stephanie with her Holly Hobbie lunchbox and Michael wearing Tom's old brown coat with fake fur around the hood. He is lost somewhere in its immensity, but because it belonged to Tom, Michael feels bigger. I remember them walking to school "together," with Michael about five paces ahead of his younger sister. I think about our lives then, and for a moment I desperately want to go back. "You can't go back," Rex's voice interrupts. But for the moment, his logic doesn't deter me.

I try to remember us—what we were like, what we thought about, the depth of our understanding. Life was good. I liked Rex being healthy and strong, even if that was something I took for granted. But when I think of us then as compared to now, I realize how much we have learned. Rex's physical body was stronger, but he now has so much more spiritual strength. He is more empathetic. His understanding of life with all of its complexities has intensified, and his faith in God has matured. He has learned patience, become more sensitive, and increased in his awareness of others.

And me? I remember myself as young and inexperienced. I was raising seven children, active in the Church, and busy with Rex's involvement with the law school as well as my own endeavors. As I look at that time more clearly, I recognize that I have grown too. I realize I have gained insights into our Savior's life and atonement, events that sustain and lift us. The challenges we have faced have brought new understanding, which I now see as an essential part of God's plan. Rex and I share a love for each other that I could not have comprehended as a starry-eyed coed, looking into Rex's warm brown eyes, or even as a young mother busy with an ever-active family.

I have come to see hope as something beyond merely wishing my husband could be well. I am not yet ready to give up that hope, but when it no longer seems possible, I will hope that he can still be with us a while longer; and when the shortness of his earthly stay is evident, I will hope for his comfort and for the strength to help him through his final moments of mortality. Then, when he is no longer here, I will hope that my life will merit my joining him some day and that I can fill the time in between with happiness, with an appreciation for my family, with a clarity of purpose, and with the strength to give service—all with much-needed steadfastness and faith in my Father in Heaven.

As I turn up the hill toward home, I realize that I have been gone for more than an hour. People are rushing to work and school, and I know I need to hurry to help Rex. Then, as I walk up the driveway toward our house, I think of the last time Rex and I ran along the Potomac River, just before his first cancer was discovered. I think of that spring morning when we laughed like children in the warm Virginia sunshine, and I am keenly aware of all the learning and all the love that have filled our lives since that day. I turn for a moment and watch the sun trying to make its way through the clouds, and

I think of all the mornings when that same sun has risen over these mountains, warming and brightening our lives and reaffirming the existence of a God in heaven who gives light and life to all the world.

With gratitude, I look back over the years, remembering the process as well as the progress. Then, with faith overshadowing my fears, I look into our unknown future and open the door. I know Rex is waiting.

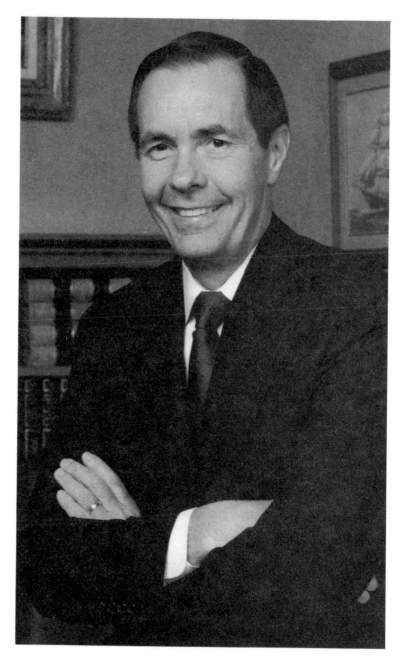

Rex Edwin Lee
February 27, 1935—March 11, 1996

Epilogue

Early on the Sunday of February 25, 1996, feeling too exhausted to attend church, Rex suggested that he could teach our Sunday School class if we held it in our home. (We had taught the seventeen- and eighteen-year-olds in our ward for several years—and we had enjoyed this calling immensely.) Rex's suggestion was characteristic of his desire to find ways to lighten my responsibilities, and on this Sunday morning, he again wanted to help in some way as he watched me prepare for our large family Sunday dinner.

Sometimes we taught our lessons together. Other times we alternated, having one teach while the other gave backup support. Lately, the job had been largely mine, with our son Michael filling in if we were out of town or Rex was in the hospital. Our class was large, somewhere between fifteen and twenty, and we were constantly amazed at the depth of these high school students' spiritual understanding. Through the years we have been pleased to have been able to have our daughters Stephanie, Melissa, and now Christie in our class.

As I brought the class into our living room, Rex was already seated in an armchair, with life-giving oxygen being provided to his damaged lungs through tubing extending to a tank in the next room. Earlier, he had asked if he needed to wear a white shirt and tie, but I knew there was great effort and some pain involved in his changing clothes, so I encouraged him to dress only once. He had opted for a more casual combination of cotton pants and a sport shirt that he could wear with comfort the rest of the day.

I watched with great admiration and love as he taught our class, asking questions, listening to responses, and praising students for their knowledge of the gospel. He spoke of the Book of Mormon, of its truthfulness, and of its application to our lives today. The last scripture I remember him quoting was "I will go and do the things which the Lord hath commanded" (1 Nephi 3:7), and I could not help but reflect that Rex, throughout his life, had always done exactly that.

When the lesson was over and the class left, I made sure that Rex was comfortable before I went to sacrament meeting. As I drove the short distance to our chapel, a melancholy feeling came over me. I thought of the struggle Rex was undergoing, how difficult it was for him to perform ordinary tasks, and how dependent he was on me to get through each day. I was willing to do anything necessary to be with him, and he pushed himself to keep going. And with each increment in the progression of his illness, he adjusted with an attitude of acceptance that was beyond my expectation of simple submission.

A year or two ago, he had dreaded the time when he could not walk, but now we were planning trips with a wheelchair and oxygen tanks with joyous anticipation. His attitude—both spoken and unspoken—was "Just let me live my life, and I will do it with whatever limitations I am given." I loved his willingness to be part of our lives for as long as possible, but I was beginning to wonder how long that would be. As I pulled up in front of the church, I sat in the car for a moment and bowed my head. A prayer I had been afraid to offer was spoken silently and somewhat reluctantly. In that moment I knew his life was in the Lord's hands—and that no matter how hard I tried to keep him here, I was not the one in control.

It was with great effort that I whispered, "Thy will be done," but peace came in knowing that while I could not comprehend all things, the loving Father to whom I had just prayed was both omniscient and omnipotent.

After our meetings, the family gathered in our home for Sunday dinner. The conversation was lively, as usual, and the grandchildren made their customary exits and entrances into our family room, outside, and downstairs in the playroom. With typical good humor, Rex visited with everyone, ate dinner with us, and was the center of attention even from his place on the couch. When he needed something, others were eager to get it for him, and when he wanted to walk a short distance, there was always someone at his side. Although his health had declined over the past several weeks, we were all used to his routine, and the day seemed quite normal. In fact, with all of the familiar activity, I found myself setting aside my earlier concerns.

Although this was a Sunday like so many others we had spent together, it was meaningful, with its beauty growing out of its simplicity. Before everyone left, our sons asked Rex if he would like them to give the sacrament to him. Tom and Michael went into the kitchen and made the proper preparation, returning to the family room where Rex remained on the couch. First, the three of them sang a hymn in Spanish. They sang with gusto in a language they all loved. Then the prayers were offered and the bread and water were administered with reverence. Following the sacrament, Tom, Michael, and Diana's husband, Steve, gave Rex a blessing. There were tears in our eyes as we all gathered for a family prayer.

We said good-bye to everyone but our two youngest children, Melissa and Christie, who remained with us for the next couple of hours until it was time for bed. The four of us were unaware that this would be our last evening with Rex in our family room. He laughed and talked with us the way we had done on so many other occasions. The girls then helped me with the difficult task of helping Rex upstairs, and we joked about wishing we could carry him piggyback the way he had conveyed the girls to their beds when they were younger. We adjusted the oxygen and then told Melissa good-bye when her husband, Brett, came to take her home. I then helped Rex get into his pajamas while Christie got ready for bed.

When she came in to say good night, Rex was lying in bed exhausted. He perked up at the sound of her voice and spoke her name to get her attention. " Christie," he said, "I just want you to know how very proud I am of you. Your participation in our Sunday School class this morning was outstanding, and I loved the way you spoke up with confidence and enthusiasm. I am so pleased that you are in our class. In fact, Christie, I am so very pleased with everything you are doing with your life. I am proud of the way you interact with your friends and family, I am proud of your performance at school, and I am very proud to be your father. I love you very much."

"I love you, too, Dad," she said as she kissed us good night.

For the next few moments in the darkness of our room, we talked happily about the U.S. Supreme Court case that Rex would argue in a few weeks and of our two new grandchildren who would be born in May and October. Then just before Rex fell asleep, I told him I had a new plan—that we should invite a few couples into our home once a week so we could enjoy being with friends without the worry of transporting oxygen. "It will be fun," I told him. "I love it when you talk that way," he said and closed his eyes.

The next morning, after months of recurring respiratory infections complicated by his cancer and progressive peripheral neuropathy, Rex was taken to the hospital the day before his sixty-first birthday. During the night, the all too familiar pattern of chills and fever had set in, and when it became clear that his need for oxygen was exceeding our home supply, we left for what was to be our last trip to the hospital together. Characteristically, he kept putting off our departure because he planned to participate in a scheduled conference call, but we finally had to leave before the call came.

For the next two weeks Rex was in the intensive care unit at the Utah Valley Regional Medical Center. The family gathered around his hospital bed, at first engaging him in conversation and, on his birthday, joining with him in a quiet celebration. Then, as his condition worsened, we simply spoke words of love and admiration. At times, our tears mingled with laughter as we remembered our favorite "Rex Lee" stories and personality traits.

For a time I felt an almost desperate need to speak with him, to hear and be heard. But as communication became difficult and then impossible, previous conversations between us played through my mind. Words unspoken now seemed insignificant and unnecessary. A lifetime of sharing had been stored in our hearts. We had found fulfillment in each other's successes and had felt sadness in our sorrows. He had helped with my challenges and rejoiced in my triumphs. Likewise, I had supported him in all that he did.

Now, in his hospital room, I thought about the many things he had been asked to do, and I was aware that what we were doing now was the most difficult of all. I tried to think of what he would tell me if he could, and then I remembered what I needed to know.

Rex's accomplishments were many, and although he didn't aspire to the positions given him, he worked hard to achieve excellence in everything he did. Each time we faced a turning point in our lives, I would ask what I could do to help. His answer was always the same and always unequivocal: "Just be happy, Janet." Now, in the midst of our final challenge, his words came back to me. Yet this previously simple request now seemed an impossibility.

For almost nine years, Rex and I had known that as his health challenges increased, we would fight for his life together. I had always promised that as living became more difficult for him, I would be there holding his hand, giving comfort, and easing his pain in any way I could. I had told him that when his mortal strength was gone, I would be strong for both of us, finding joy in loving life as we had always done together. I would see him in each of our children and grandchildren, I would be reminded of him in every season, and I would feel close to him each time I bowed my head in gratitude to our Father in Heaven. I would run and think of him, and when I became too old to run, I would walk and imagine him by my side. I had offered these promises effortlessly and lovingly. But I had never considered happiness as part of the process of letting go.

On Monday, March eleventh, we knew that Rex's earthly life was coming to a close. Our seven children joined me in his hospital room as we spoke of favorite shared experiences, of our love for him, and of our faith in God. The last outpouring of our hearts paid tribute to our husband and father. Then, as efficiently and purposefully as he had lived his life, surrounded by our eternal family and with his hand in mine, Rex left mortality. As I held him close, I was filled with appreciation for the life we had shared. I felt his spirit soar as I whispered words of love and gratitude. I knew he was free from his pain, and I could feel his joy. Unexpectedly, the sharing of his triumph subdued my personal sadness as I said, "I am so happy for you, Sweetheart."

Together we had run many miles, loving life, raising our children, confronting illness, expressing our love for each other and for our Savior, and preparing for the day that we knew would come too soon. As I walked out of the hospital that afternoon, his words filled my heart: "Just be happy, Janet."

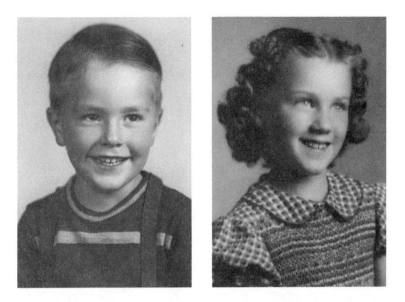

Rex Lee and Janet Griffin in their younger years

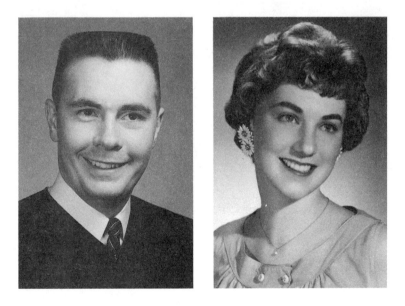

Rex and Janet in the mid-1950s

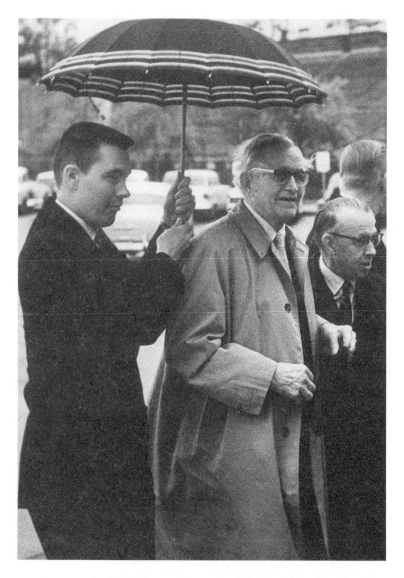

As BYU student body president in 1960,
Rex accompanies President David O. McKay and
BYU President Ernest L. Wilkinson to a devotional assembly
in the Smith Fieldhouse.

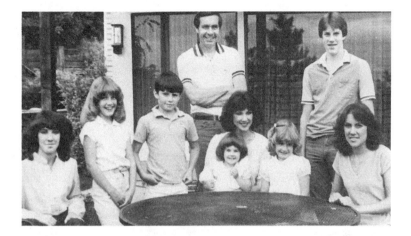

IN 1979, THE LEE FAMILY INCLUDES (LEFT TO RIGHT) WENDY, STEPHANIE, MICHAEL, REX, JANET, CHRISTIE (ON JANET'S LAP), MELISSA, TOM, AND DIANA.

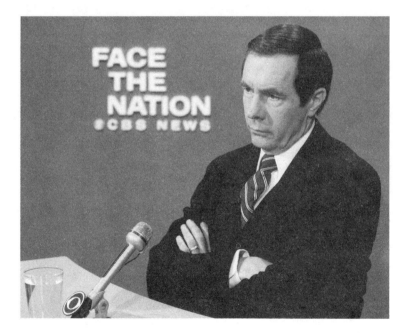

AS UNITED STATES SOLICITOR GENERAL DURING THE REAGAN ADMINISTRATION, REX E. LEE IS CALLED UPON FREQUENTLY TO COMMENT ON CASES BEING TAKEN TO THE NATION'S HIGHEST COURT.

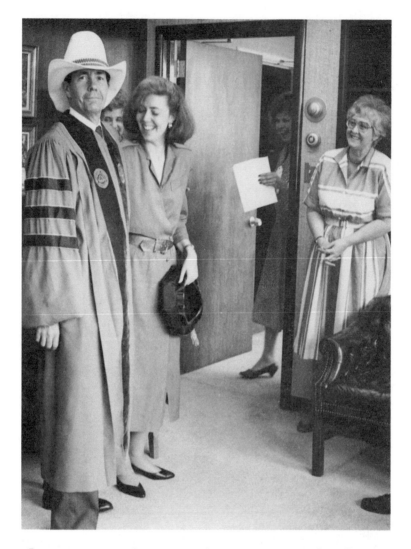

REX CHATTING WITH (LEFT TO RIGHT) STUDENT ASSISTANT CHAR TANNER
AND HIS TWO SECRETARIES, JAN NELSON AND JANET CALDER, PRIOR TO
A FULL DAY AND NIGHT OF INAUGURAL ACTIVITIES

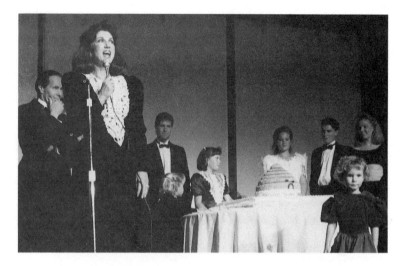

JANET GREETS WELL-WISHERS AT THE LEES' INAUGURAL BALL.

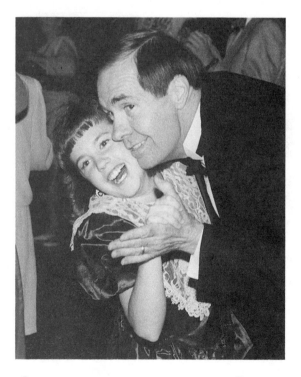

REX ENJOYS A DANCE WITH HIS DAUGHTER CHRISTIE
DURING HIS INAUGURAL BALL.

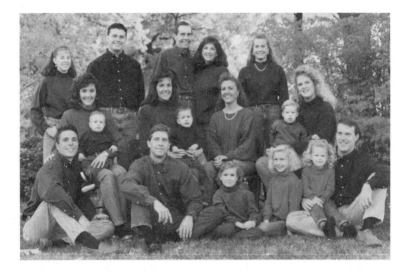

THE REX AND JANET LEE FAMILY
IN 1992

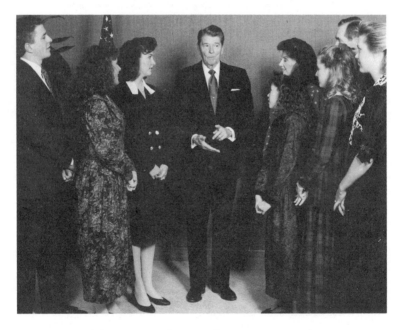

FORMER U.S. PRESIDENT RONALD REAGAN WITH THE LEE FAMILY
DURING HIS 1991 VISIT TO BYU

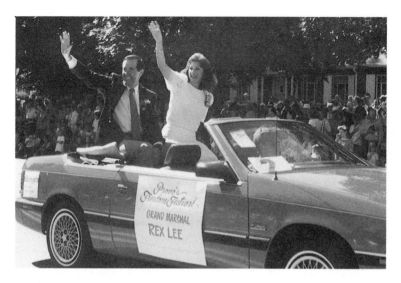

REX AND JANET AT PROVO'S FOURTH OF JULY CELEBRATION

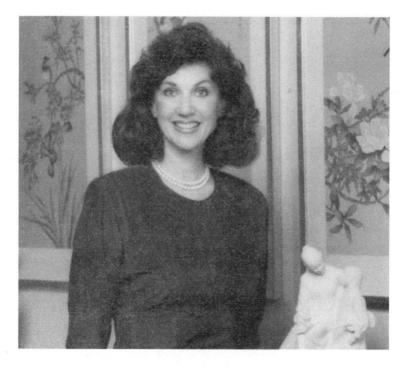

JANET GRIFFIN LEE, SOON AFTER REX'S APPOINTMENT AS PRESIDENT
OF BRIGHAM YOUNG UNIVERSITY

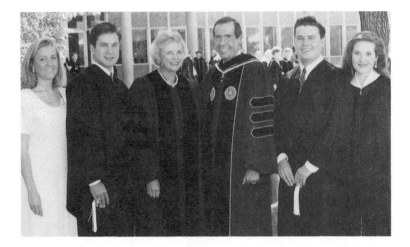

AT BYU'S AUGUST 1994 COMMENCEMENT, REX IS JOINED
BY HIS LONGTIME FRIEND SANDRA DAY O'CONNOR, AS WELL AS HIS
DAUGHTER STEPHANIE LEE PAULSON (FAR LEFT) AND THREE GRADUATES
FROM THE FAMILY—BRET PAULSON, MICHAEL, AND MICHAEL'S WIFE,
SHARON BURR LEE.

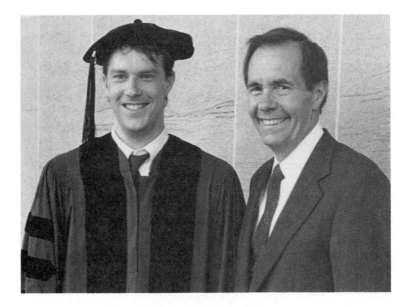

REX JOINS HIS SON TOM AT THE TIME OF TOM'S GRADUATION
FROM THE UNIVERSITY OF CHICAGO LAW SCHOOL.

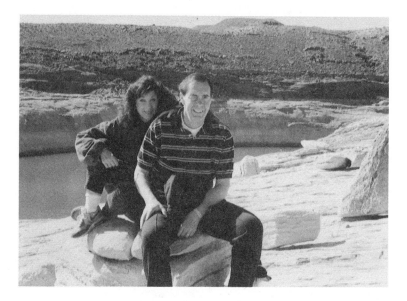

REX AND JANET ENJOY A MOMENT TOGETHER
DURING A FAMILY VACATION TO LAKE POWELL.

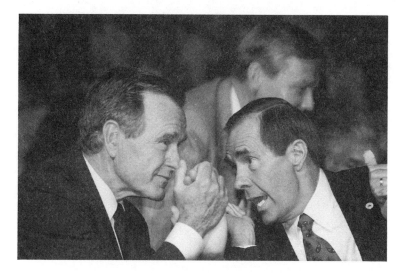

PRESIDENT LEE VISITS WITH PRESIDENT GEORGE BUSH
DURING HIS VISIT TO BYU IN 1992.

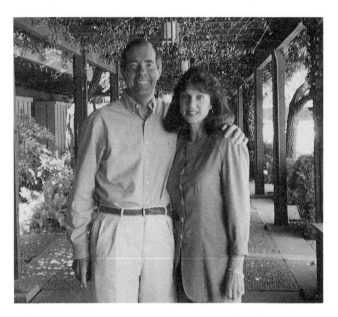

REX AND JANET RELAX TOGETHER IN CARMEL, CALIFORNIA, IN 1994.

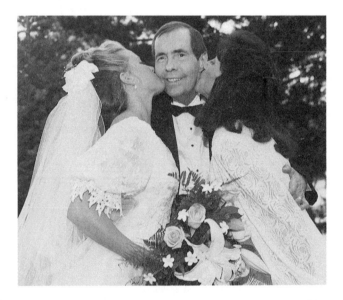

THE FATHER OF THE BRIDE ENJOYS A KISS FROM HIS DAUGHTER, MELISSA,
AND THE MOTHER OF THE BRIDE, AUGUST 1995.